The Doctor's Guide to Milk and Your Health

The Good, the Bad or the Slow Poison

Anil Minocha, MD

Professor of Medicine

Fellow, American College of Physicians

Fellow, American College of Gastroenterology

Fellow, American Gastroenterological Association

Other Books by Dr. Minocha

Is it Leaky Gut or Leaky Gut Syndrome?

Dr. M's Seven-X Plan for Digestive Health

A Guide to Alternative System and the Digestive System

Encyclopedia of Digestive System and Digestive Disorders

Handbook of Digestive Diseases

Natural Stomach Care

Copyright

ISBN: 978-0-9915031-4-8

Library of Congress Control Number:
2015920805

Disclaimer

The publisher has put forth its best efforts in preparing and arranging this book. The information provided herein by the author is provided "as is" and you read and use this information at your own risk. The publisher and author disclaim any liabilities for any loss of profit or commercial or personal damages resulting from the use of the information contained in this book.

This work is meant for informational use only and by no means represents recommendations for diagnosis or treatment of any disorder for any reader. Neither the publisher nor the author is engaged in rendering medical advice or services to any individual reader. Nothing in this book is intended to be a substitute for consultation with a licensed physician. All matters of health require medical supervision. The book is meant to provide you with information so you may make your own decisions. Only your licensed medical provider can determine what diet and remedies are in the best interest of your health and what to do about your illness. Never implement any health information from a book without discussing it with your physician.

The procedures, treatments, and practices described in this book should be implemented only by a licensed physician and only in a manner consistent with the professional standards set for the circumstances that apply to each specific situation. Neither the publisher nor the author is responsible for your specific health or allergy needs that may require medical attention. The author, editor, and publisher cannot accept responsibility for errors, exclusions, or the outcome of the application of the material presented herein. There is no expressed or implied warranty of this book or the information imparted by it.

Neither the publisher nor the author has financial interest in the pharmaceuticals, over-the-counter medications including supplements, or any medical equipment mentioned in this book.

Please note that the book was previously beta-tested in published format using another title for a few days.

If you enjoyed this book, please encourage your friends to get their own copy.

Preface

I think we ought always to entertain our opinions with some measure of doubt. I shouldn't wish people dogmatically to believe any philosophy, not even mine.

---Bertrand Russell

Medicine is an art, not a science, and our already vast knowledge is increasing exponentially. This book fulfils the need for a quick, concise source of practical information, allowing the reader to better understand the concept and controversies surrounding the use of milk and be a better-informed consumer of health information, especially during a visit to the physician.

To achieve the goal of providing a condensed version of the state of knowledge for a broad audience, I have presented the current findings in literature as well as controversial positions. As in most cases of medical science, everyone has an opinion. Knowledge that was deemed to be an indisputable fact only a few years ago may now be cast away as rubbish. Just take an example of fats, including saturated fats, which are no longer considered to be as bad as was taught and practiced for decades! Bacteria in the stomach have now been confirmed to be a major cause of ulcers, even though the concept of infection-causing ulcers had been dismissed for decades as an old wives' tale.

I am of the opinion that our digestive system and nutrition play a critical role in health and sickness. This is not a new concept. Hippocrates thought of the same thing thousands of years ago when he stated, "*All diseases begin in the gut.*"

In fact, our gut has a brain of its own and the term "gut psychology" has been used to describe the role of the gut in anxiety and depression.

I have at times in this book, sacrificed finer detail and nuances for the sake of brevity and clarity. This book should not be used to make a diagnosis or initiate any treatment. All illness requires medical supervision by a licensed physician. And yes, I have had my own health challenges in life. That is all the more reason for me to share what I have learned both professionally and personally over the years.

Towards the end, I have provided a bonus section that includes a chapter each from a couple of my other books highlighting the significance of gut and nutrition in overall health and sickness.

Knowledge is broad-based, and each person is unique. It is critical that no one adopt any changes based on this book or for that matter any other book without discussing them with a physician.

I wish all my readers a happy and healthy life.

Table of Contents

Section 1

Primer on Milk

CHAPTER 1

Introduction

Milk is a very generic term used for a variety of products from various sources currently available on market. The term milk when used in commercial sense refers mostly to cow's milk unless otherwise specified, for example, soy milk, almond milk etc. Milk from other animals like sheep and goat milk are also available on the market.

NO MILK IS PERFECT INCLUDING MOM'S

Mom's milk meets the nutritional needs of babies for six months, except for vitamins D and K. In fact, breastfed infants may benefit from an injection of vitamin K and should receive vitamin D supplementation.

Human milk is low in docosahexaenoic acid (DHA), so supplementation may be needed for babies exclusively breastfed for prolonged periods.

Maternal diet varies which affects the composition of breast milk. As such, it is prudent for lactating moms to take multivitamin-mineral supplements.

HUMAN CONSUMPTION OF COW'S MILK

Cow's milk has become part of our staple diet based on our culture and traditions. But has it become a problem in recent decades, at least more so in the developed countries?

- While many of us may be able to handle cow's milk reasonably well, certain people at risk may be harmed. Individuals at risk include:

- Those with unhealthy genes.

- Those with a deficiency of digestive enzymes, which does not allow the gut to break down the relative high amounts of proteins like casein.

- Those with leaky gut, which allows passage of larger, semi-digested breakdown products of milk proteins across the gut wall into the body.

It is not necessarily always the natural cow's milk at fault. The processing of cow's milk has been incriminated as the source of idiopathic membranous nephropathy in some children.

The potentially adverse impact of cow's milk may in part be a function of "unnatural" alterations in the cow's milk produced by a variety of methods used to increase the amount of milk produced.

According to Dr. Wiley from the Human Biology Program and Department of Anthropology, Indiana University, Bloomington, Indiana, *"Routine milk consumption is an evolutionarily novel dietary behavior that has the potential to alter human life history parameters...which in turn may have negative long-term biological consequences"*.

Above notwithstanding, Kliem and Givens conclude, based on the totality of evidence, that people with a higher intake of milk and dairy products may have a slightly better health profile as compared to those who completely avoid them. However, remember, statistics do not always apply to individuals. Each person is unique in his/her genetic and metabolic profile as well as in their susceptibility to physical impairments and mental dysfunction.

REFERENCES

1. Agostoni C, Decsi T, Fewtrell M, Goulet O et al. ESPGHAN Committee on Nutrition:. Complementary feeding: a commentary by the ESPGHAN Committee on Nutrition. J Pediatr Gastroenterol Nutr. 2008 Jan;46(1):99-110.

2. Ghisolfi J, Fantino M, Turck D, de Courcy GP, Vidailhet M. Nutrient intakes of children aged 1-2 years as a function of milk consumption, cows' milk or growing-up milk. Public Health Nutr. 2013 Mar;16(3):524-34.

3. Kliem KE, Givens DI. Dairy products in the food chain: their impact on health. Annu Rev Food Sci Technol. 2011;2:21-36.

4. Wiley AS. Cow milk consumption, insulin-like growth factor-I, and human

biology: a life history approach. Am J
Hum Biol. 2012 Mar-Apr;24(2):130-8.

CHAPTER 2

A Historical and Evolutionary Journey

According to Oftedal from the Smithsonian Environmental Research Center, as published in the journal *Animal*, the evolutionary origin of milk goes back to its secretion from the skin glands about 310 million years ago. In fact, the origin of nutritious milk may predate the origin of mammals.

THE ORIGIN OF MAMMARY GLANDS

The mammary glands likely arose from skin glands along with the hair follicles. Along the way, different defensive components of milk, both nutritious and non-nutritious, came into use for sustenance of the helpless baby.

Changes in digestive enzymes and bioactive metabolic compounds came about as a result of the evolution of new types of sugars.

Genes for milk, mammary glands and lactation have been remarkably conserved during the course of evolution, more than any other mammalian genes indicating the importance of milk to both mother and off spring.

THE TRIASSIC PERIOD

During the late Triassic period (200-250 million years ago), milk replaced egg as the primary source of nutrition for newborns. However, the framework of milk, with its main fats and proteins, occurred prior to the appearance of mammals. Thus, the roots of the milk industry were established long before the dinosaur era.

THE NEOLITHIC REVOLUTION

Dairying started along with plant cultivation, animals farming and numerous other socio-economic changes. Female animals were preferentially kept alive longer than the male counterparts who were slaughtered for meat.

Evidence suggests gene-culture co-evolution with the active persistence of lactase enzyme and the dairy breeding.

MODERN MILK

Modern milk owes its origin to the continued changes in milk and mammary genes over the course of evolution, allowing for selection and conservation of beneficial genes based on different needs of the evolving species.

REFERENCES

1. Oftedal OT. The evolution of milk secretion and its ancient origins. Animal. 2012 Mar;6(3):355-68.

2. Lefèvre CM, Sharp JA, Nicholas KR. Evolution of lactation: ancient origin and extreme adaptations of the lactation system. Annu Rev Genomics Hum Genet. 2010;11:219-38.

3. Gerbault P, Roffet-Salque M, Evershed RP, Thomas MG. How long have adult humans been consuming milk? IUBMB Life. 2013 Dec;65(12):983-90.

CHAPTER 3

Milk: The First Food for Mammals

Before we start, let us just stipulate that, irrespective of the source, milk is full of nutritious components. Let us also stipulate that cow's milk overall has served as a good source of nutrition to humans over thousands of years.

Cow's milk has been recommended as an essential component of the everyday adult diet by health authorities for decades. It is a good source of proteins, vitamins, and minerals. In fact, dairy and dairy products are an important component of the *MyPlate* menu recommended by the Centers for Diseases Control (CDC).

MILK AND THE LACTATION PROCESS

Milk is a biologic fluid that is a unique feature of mammals. Unlike the standardized formula feed, biologic milk is a dynamic fluid that changes to meet the needs of the baby as it grows.

Milk produced at the time of birth is not the same as the milk produced when the baby is one week old. Nature created milk as a maternal lactating secretion, a nutrient and defense complex, for the newborn during its most vulnerable period of life. Subsequently, as the baby's own defenses come to fruition, the weaning process occurs.

MILK IS JUST NOT FOOD

Milk is not just a source of energy or simply building blocks for growth and development. In fact, it is naïve to assume of the consumption of milk merely in terms of energy consumption. It should be noted that the health and nutritional implications of milk are not the same as for fermented milk.

BIOLOGICAL FUNCTIONS

Milk plays an important role in immune health, especially during the early vulnerable period of life. Milk proteins can act as enzymes, antibacterial agents, and hormones.

Many breakdown products of milk proteins have biological functions such as the modification of the immune system, enzyme systems, and platelets. In fact, while continued use of cow's milk has been implicated in some adverse long-term health consequences, recent literature also suggests that milk contains many important biologically-active compounds that have the potential to decrease risk of many such diseases. The key is in being able to harness these health promoting compounds for use on mass scale.

MILK AS A MOM-TO-BABY COMMUNICATION SYSTEM

According to *Dr. Melnik* and colleagues from the University of Osnabrück, Germany, milk is a materno-neonatal relay system functioning by transfer of preferential amino acids from mother to the baby. This chemical communication system plays a critical role in activating a variety of hormones, including growth hormones in the baby.

MILK EXOSOMES CONTAIN CHEMICAL SIGNALS

Like other bodily fluids, milk also naturally contains exosomes. These are tiny vesicles lined by specialized membranes derived from components of the cells. These exosomes contain a variety of substances and act as signals between cells. Initially condemned as mostly garbage cans, the discovery of genetic material in these exosomes has intensified scientific interest.

MILK AS A GENETIC TRANSFECTION SYSTEM

Milk exosomes contain genetic material. As such, these represent a genetic transfection organisation whose purpose is to stimulate various processes of metabolism in the growing baby. It thus stands to reason that mom's breast milk would be the most perfect food for baby since it permits growth befitting humans along with human-specific metabolic programming during early childhood. Some experts theorize that continued high cow milk consumption past adolescence and into adulthood may increase risk for certain metabolically-driven diseases of civilization.

ARE EXOSOMES PRESENT IN COMMERCIAL COW'S MILK?

Indeed they are!

Dr. Pieters and colleagues from the Radboud University Medical Centre in Nijmegen, the Netherlands, isolated and characterized extracellular vesicles present in semi-skimmed cow milk available for consumers. They then studied the effects of these exosomes on immune cells. These investigators demonstrated that milk exosomes are very stable and resistant to boiling or freezing. They contain genetic material in the form of RNA as well as specialized bioactive proteins and antibodies.

Above results indicate that exosomes in commercial bovine milk do not get degraded in the gut but rather, promote immune-regulatory effects. As such, it has the potential to affect health and sickness especially when milk is consumed life-long unlike, any other species.

REFERENCES

1. Melnik BC, John SM, Schmitz G. Milk is not just food but most likely a genetic transfection system activating mTORC1 signaling for postnatal growth. *Nutr J.* 2013 Jul 25;12:103.

2. Pieters BC, Arntz OJ, Bennink MB, Broeren MG et al. Commercial Cow Milk Contains Physically Stable Extracellular Vesicles Expressing Immunoregulatory TGF-β. *PLoS One.* 2015 Mar 30;10(3):e0121123.

CHAPTER 4

Changes in Recent Times

GENES VERSUS ENVIRONMENT

Our core genes have stayed relatively stable, with some mutations or epigenetic phenomenon along the way, over tens of thousands of years of evolution.

ROLE OF EPIGENETICS

The mere presence of a gene does not mean that it is functionally active. Genes are present in the cells. However, they can be in an active or inactive state. As such, while structurally the gene may be present, but functionally silent, it might as well be absent for all intents and purposes.

Epigenetics is the study of changes in the functioning of the genes as a result of environmental factors (such as diet or toxins).

Changes in gene functioning may involve turning the gene "on" or "off." These functional changes can be genetically passed on to the next generation of the animal. An example of non-genetic influences affecting the functioning of genes is the cessation of milk secretion when the breasts are inflamed and/or infected, or as the breasts shrink.

Other cow-related factors with the potential to affect gene functioning include human impacts such as on tight living conditions, use of hormones, and antibiotics etc.

WE HAVE CHANGED, AS HAS OUR ENVIRONMENT

Ancient humans lived as part of nature as 'hunter-gatherers.' We now have a fast-paced world with higher environmental pollution, and a relatively sedentary lifestyle.

It is not surprising that our genes are not functioning the same way as they did in ancient times, when human beings actually had to hunt for food rather than just driving to the supermarket.

THE COWS HAVE CHANGED

Even the cows don't drink the cow's milk we do. Cows drink milk from free-living cows, while we drink milk from caged animals. The cow's milk consumed by humans is not "natural" due to many factors:

- Specialized and selective breeding.

- Use of assisted reproductive technologies to increase the production of dairy cattle. The in vitro produced cow embryos are very different from their natural counterparts in many facets, including developmental competence.

- Use of herd management programs to increase bovine fertility which in turn increases overall milk production.

- Use of unnatural methods to increase reproductivity including but not limited to timed artificial insemination.

- Use of artificial climatic conditions to enable increased milk production and reproduction.

- Increasing exposure of cows to electrical currents/voltage in farms.

- Overall unnatural living conditions.

- Use of drugs and hormones administered to the cows to increase milk yield.

- Use of antibiotics given to cows for frequent infections.

Holstein cattle are being bred increasingly and selectively in an effort to meet the increasing milk demands of the populace. Holstein comprise 90% of the cow species subtype in the U.S. and 85% in the United Kingdom. In India, most of the milk is home-delivered especially in villages. Thus the quality of milk can vary from region to region.

RUSH TO INCREASE MILK PRODUCTION TO MEET DEMANDS

The average herd size in developed countries has increased dramatically in recent years, as has the annual milk production per cow. Dairy cattle are now bred with the primary purpose of increasing milk production.

Cows in Israeli dairy farms produce 12,546 kg of milk per year, compared to cows in New Zealand, which yield 4,100 kg per year. The factors affecting the yield include production systems and cows' diet. For example, most cows in New Zealand graze freely all year; in Israel, the cows are fed an energy-rich mixed diet in closed quarters.

Cow's milk itself cannot be the sole factor causing problems in humans. A genetic vulnerability is critical, along with many other factors, including pollution and potentially other toxins consumed in diet.

REFERENCES

1. Singh K, Molenaar AJ, Swanson KM, Gudex B et al. Epigenetics: a possible role in acute and transgenerational regulation of dairy cow milk production. *Animal*. 2012 Mar;6(3):375-81.

2. Kyselková M, Jirout J, Vrchotová N, Schmitt H, Elhottová D. Spread of tetracycline resistance genes at a conventional dairy farm. *Front Microbiol*. 2015 May 29;6:536.

3. Bargo F, Muller LD, Kolver ES, Delahoy JE. Invited review: production and digestion of supplemented dairy cows on pasture. J Dairy Sci. 2003 Jan;86(1):1-42.

4. Schwendel BH, Morel PC, Wester TJ, Tavendale MH et al. Fatty acid profile differs between organic and conventionally produced cow milk independent of season or milking time. *J Dairy Sci*. 2015 Mar;98(3):1411-25.

5. Aguilar M, Hanigan MD, Tucker HA, Jones BL et al. Cow and herd variation in milk urea nitrogen concentrations in lactating dairy cattle. *J Dairy Sci*. 2012 Dec;95(12):7261-8.

6. Cabrera VE. Economics of fertility in high-yielding dairy cows on confined TMR systems. *Animal*. 2014 May;8 Suppl 1:211-21.

7. McDougall S, Heuer C, Morton J, Brownlie T. Use of herd management programmes to improve the reproductive performance of dairy cattle. *Animal*. 2014 May;8 Suppl1:199-210.

8. Flamenbaum I, Galon N. Management of heat stress to improve fertility in dairy cows in Israel. *J Reprod Dev*. 2010 Jan;56 Suppl:S36-41.

CHAPTER 5

Composition of Milk

Milk, regardless of the species, has major macro-nutrients as well as micro-nutrients. Human milk contains about 12 g of protein, 35 g of fat and 70 g of lactose per liter. While the protein content of the milk (colostrum) when the baby is born is as high as 2.3%, the mature human milk is just 1% protein.

This chapter deals with the composition of milk in general and human milk in particular. The specific differences between human milk and cow's milk and the potential superiority of human milk tailored to human needs are discussed in subsequent chapters.

PROTEINS

Milk proteins are mainly comprised of caseins and whey. The proportion of various proteins in the milk varies by species and breed. These proteins are digested in the gut into smaller components for absorption. For any species, the higher the protein content, the faster the baby can double its weight.

WHEY PROTEINS

Whey has been recognized as beneficial since ancient times. An ancient proverb states, *"If everyone was raised on whey, doctors would be bankrupt."*

Whey protein complex includes alfa-lactalbumin, lactoferrin, antibodies, lysozyme, and albumin.

There are remarkable differences in whey proteins present in milk of humans and other species, both with respect to the total proportion as well as individual components like alpha-lactalbumin, lactoferrin, antibodies etc.

CASEINS

The total amount and types of caseins in milk are also different among the species. Most mammalian milk has three or four types of caseins. Caseins form only about 40 % of the total human protein.

Dr. Fiat has described a *"strategic zone"* occurs among caseins containing immune-stimulating and opioid peptides.

Studies by Dr. Tanabe and colleagues suggest that protein breakdown products (peptides) derived from the digestion of casein in the human milk can strengthen the intestinal barrier, reinforcing the importance of breastfeeding for growth and immune defenses of the baby.

Since the biologically active casein proteins are different in different species, they may be beneficial to the baby of that species, but potentially harmful when consumed by another species.

SUPERIORITY OF HUMAN MILK PROTEINS

The proteins in human milk are balanced and more fine-tuned to human digestive and absorption processes. This meets the baby's unique protein requirements commensurate with healthy growth and development while protecting the baby's immature kidneys from an overload of protein waste.

CARBOHYDRATES

Carbohydrates in milk are mainly composed of lactose. In addition, human milk also provides 10 grams per liter of non-digestible oligosaccharides. These act as prebiotics and promote the growth of beneficial protective gut bacteria in the infant.

FATS

Fat content of human milk is 3.9 %. While the difference in total fat content is not too wide among higher mammalian species, there are marked differences in the fatty acid and triglyceride composition. This has huge implications for relative differences in the development of nervous system between different species.

FATTY ACIDS

Saturated fatty acids (1.9 %) are thought to contribute to heart disease, increased cholesterol, and obesity although the thinking in this respect is evolving. In addition, not all saturated fatty acids are bad. Some of these saturated fatty acids, like butyric acid, may actually be beneficial for health as well.

- Breastfed infants have a higher concentration of docosahexaenoic acid (DHA) than formula-fed infants. Studies by Dr. Gale and colleagues indicate that children fed breast milk or DHA-fortified formula during infancy have higher full-scale and verbal I.Q. scores by the age of four years, compared to those fed unfortified formula.

- A mother's consumption of cod liver oil, which contains important fatty acids, improves her child's I.Q., compared to moms provided with a corn-oil supplementation. This suggests that mother's milk is better than formula in providing key nutrients in a balanced fashion for optimal development of the brain.

REFERENCES

1. Pereira PC. Milk nutritional composition and its role in human health. Nutrition. 2014 Jun;30(6):619-27.

2. Krissansen GW. Emerging health properties of whey proteins and their clinical implications. J Am Coll Nutr. 2007 Dec; 26(6):713S-23S.

3. Zhang Z, Adelman AS, Rai D et al. Amino Acid Profiles in Term and Preterm Human Milk through Lactation: A Systematic Review. Nutrients. 2013 Nov 26;5(12):4800-21.

4. Hsieh CC, Hernández-Ledesma B, Fernández-Tomé S et al. Milk proteins, peptides, and oligosaccharides: effects against the 21st century disorders. Biomed Res Int. 2015;2015:146840.

5. Fiat AM, Jollès P. Caseins of various origins and biologically active casein peptides and oligosaccharides: structural and physiological aspects. Mol Cell Biochem. 1989 May 4;87(1):5-30.

6. Tanabe S. Short peptide modules for enhancing intestinal barrier function. Curr Pharm Des. 2012;18(6):776-81.

7. Gale CR, Marriott LD, Martyn CN et al. Group for Southampton Women's Survey Study. Breastfeeding, the use of docosahexaenoic acid-fortified formulas in infancy and neuropsychological function in childhood. Arch Dis Child. 2010 Mar;95(3):174-9.

Section 11

The Milk Conundrum

CHAPTER 6

All Milk is *Not* the Same

The composition of human milk is different depending upon the time of day, age of the baby, mother's diet, race, and ethnicity. Likewise, all cow's milk is not the same. Composition of cow's milk depends on breed, season, living conditions, and type of feed etc.

- Non-nutritive bioactive factors present in a mother's milk include:

- Growth factors to promote growth and development

- Maternal immune cells

- Antibodies

- Antimicrobial chemicals to fight against infections

- Erythropoietin to support blood formation

- Prebiotic oligosaccharides to promote beneficial gut bacteria

SPECIES-SPECIFIC MAMMALIAN MILK

Milk of each mammal is unique and intended to meet the needs of the newborn of each species.

We should not just look at the macronutrient composition of milk, but also micronutrients and the relative proportions. Looking at cow's milk through this prism, it is clear and not surprising that cow's milk is simply not designed for humans. For example, cow's milk has certain blood components, albeit in small amounts, with the potential to cause problems in at-risk individuals.

Without going into too many details, suffice it to say that sheep milk is very rich in proteins and fats whereas goat milk has high concentrations of vitamins and minerals like calcium and phosphorus as compared to cow's milk.

The differences can be in immune components as well. The antibodies in camel milk are very small, about 1/10th the size of human antibodies. These have been termed nano-antibodies. These very small antibodies which after ingestion, have potential to enter across the gut barrier into the human body and consequently have an impact on human immune balance.

Above notwithstanding, the focus of the book is primarily on cow's milk although references to other sources would be made as needed.

MILK PROTEINS

In contrast to the 1% protein in human milk, cow's milk has 3.4% protein. Thus, cow's milk has a much higher level of proteins designed to help more with skeletal and muscular growth than human milk.

WHEY PROTEINS

There are remarkable differences between cow and human milk with respect to the whey proteins. The level of alpha-lactalbumin in human milk is twice as high as in cow's milk.

CASEIN PROTEINS

As discussed earlier, the total amount and types of caseins are also different between the species. Caseins form only about 40 % of the total human protein. In contrast, as much as 84% of cow's milk proteins are made up of caseins.

Since caseins and their breakdown products can have biological actions in the nervous system, a different amount and type of such caseins has potential to alter the functioning of brain.

MISCELLANEOUS BIOLOGICALLY ACTIVE PROTEIN COMPONENTS

Human milk has high concentrations of lactoferrin, an important anti-bacterial and anti-inflammatory multi-functional protein, which also stimulates cell growth. Lactoferrin is present in cow's milk in only minimal amounts.

The total antibody levels in human milk are much higher than the cow's milk. In addition, these antibodies in human milk are more specific to humans.

CARBOHYDRATES

Human milk has much higher lactose than cow's milk (6.6 % versus 4.8 %). The composition can even differ between different breeds of cows and can have significant impact on health.

For example, Dr. Sundekilde and co-investigators have shown that different breeds of cows produce milk with different amounts of oligosaccharides. Oligosaccharides in milk function as prebiotics and play significant role in the health of the baby by promoting the selective growth of beneficial bacteria in the gut. These beneficial gut bacteria in turn can have impact on immune regulation in the baby during early formative years with profound consequences for health long past childhood.

FATS

Fat content of human milk is 3.9%, compared to 3.7% in cow's milk.

FATTY ACIDS

Human milk has a much higher concentration of important essential fatty acids critical to human health as compared to cow's milk.

Long chain fatty acids play a critical role in the development of nervous system, and retina of the eyes etc. Cow's milk has more short-chain and saturated fatty acids and very few long-chain polyunsaturated fatty acids as compared to human milk. In fact, cow's milk has only about 0.2 % polyunsaturated fatty acids.

Human milk is not just a source of energy for the baby. Humans have a highly developed nervous system, and the milk fed to human babies must be commensurate to the growth and development of this nervous system relative to the musculoskeletal system.

MERITS OF DRINKING COW'S MILK

Cow's milk is a near-complete source of nutrition for the human body. It is rich in calcium, phosphorus, and vitamin D. Among animal sources of nutrition, cow's milk is perhaps one of the most economical sources of protein and many micronutrients. It serves as a valuable means for prevention and treatment of malnutrition in developing countries.

Besides the obvious nutritional benefit, there are other bioactive ingredients as well. For example, some protein components in cow's milk lower blood pressure. This is clinically corroborated by the clinical data suggesting lower incidence of high blood pressure (hypertension) among people drinking milk.

NUTRITIONAL DEFICITS OF COW'S MILK

The use of cow's milk is constantly reported in the press as well as peer-reviewed journals with respect to its potential association with iron deficiency anemia, lactose intolerance, diabetes, and many neurobehavioral disorders.

Perhaps one of the biggest nutritional deficits is low iron content. To make things worse, cow's milk prevents absorption of iron in the human baby. The iron deficit in those consuming cow's milk exclusively may be exacerbated by occult (hidden) bleeding from the gut, seen in as many as 40% of babies fed with cow's milk.

DIFFERENT FUNCTIONAL EFFECTS OF DIFFERENT TYPES OF MILK

HUMAN MILK VERSUS COW'S MILK VERSUS DONKEY MILK

Variations in components from milk derived from different animal species can have variable effects on energy utilization in the body. This has consequences for body composition and body shape and habitus via effects on mitochondria as well as on inflammation via, in part, their effect on intestinal bacteria.

Some experts consider donkey milk to be the best substitute for mother's milk in humans.

Dr. Trinchese and colleagues conducted a comparative study of the effect of equal caloric amounts of milk derived from humans, cows and donkeys on net caloric status, oxidant-antioxidant status as well as gut bacteria in rats for 4 weeks.

Results indicated that rats fed cow's milk had greater increase in weight and body fat while those fed donkey or human milk were similar to controls. Blood glucose levels were better controlled in those fed human or donkey milk. The markers of inflammation were increased in animals fed cow's milk and not others suggesting cow's milk has components that promote inflammation. In contrast, the human and donkey milk improved antioxidant status of the experimental rats in the study.

Intestinal bacteria in the rats in this study were also different. The bacterial pattern in rats fed human or donkey milk shifted towards the types of bacteria that are associated with anti-inflammatory properties and this was associated with a decrease in markers of inflammation.

Short chain fatty acids (SCFA) serve as food for the colon and their levels depend in part on the type of bacteria in the gut. Rats fed human or donkey milk showed higher levels of SCFA as compared to those consuming cow's milk further demonstrating the superiority of donkey milk over cow's milk.

So if you have to choose between cow's milk and donkey's milk for the baby, should the winner be donkey milk? You decide.

GOAT MILK

Goat's milk has less lactose than bovine milk and bears many similarities to human milk. Oligosaccharides that can act as prebiotics are not only the highest in goat's milk amongst domestic animals; they are also structurally similar to the ones seen in human milk.

Many believe that goat's milk is easier to digest by infants especially those with health problems. The jury is out on this issue.

Goat's milk contains more protein and calcium than cow's milk. On the other hand, its sugar content is less.

Goat's milk is an excellent source of protein for the baby.

Exclusive use of unmodified goat's milk as an energy source may not be appropriate for infants. While it may be safe in many children with a cow's milk allergy, it is controversial whether goat's milk offers substantial nutritional superiority over cow's milk or has overall, less of an allergenic potential.

CROSS ALLERGENICITY OF MILK FROM DIFFERENT ANIMALS

There is cross-reactivity and allergenicity between cow's milk and the milk from other mammals. It should however be noted that some children may be allergic to cow's milk but not to sheep or goat's milk. At the same time, some babies may be allergic to goat and sheep milk without exhibiting any allergy to cow's milk.

WHY DO WE DRINK COW'S MILK?

Cow's milk is a great source of nutrition, especially in developing countries. It has been a life saver for children in poor countries. For the rest of us, while we drink cow's milk based on culture and tradition, is it wise and healthy to drink cow's milk, particularly beyond childhood?

There is a good reason why the milk of every animal is distinct and naturally designed to fulfill the needs of that particular species. Just look at a cow. Does the cow bear any similarity to the human in size, height, musculoskeletal structure, or intelligence?

Risks of any deleterious action depend upon the intensity of the interactions of the toxin with the health status of the genes in any particular individual. Examination of large epidemiologic studies suggests that benefits of cow's milk consumption may outweigh potential risks in the developing countries. It saves lives!

Does the same risk-benefit concept hold true in a well-fed, fast-paced western society consuming milk produced from cows living in vastly different, and some would argue, unhealthy conditions including using antibiotics to increase production of milk?

Is it really plausible that it was God's evolutionary plan for one species to consume milk from another? If indeed it was the intention for us to drink cow's milk, would the milk from all species – or at least the cow and the human – not be similar? While it may be good for many people in certain circumstances, it may not be good for all.

REFERENCES

1. Trinchese G, Cavaliere G, Canani RB, Matamoros S et al. Human, donkey and cow milk differently affects energy efficiency and inflammatory state by modulating mitochondrial function and gut microbiota. *J Nutr Biochem*. 2015 Jun 9. pii: S0955-2863(15)00136-9.

2. Sundekilde UK, Barile D, Meyrand M, Poulsen NA et al. Natural variability in bovine milk oligosaccharides from Danish Jersey and Holstein-Friesian breeds. *J Agric Food Chem*. 2012 Jun 20;60(24):6188-96.

3. Zivkovic AM, Barile D. Bovine milk as a source of functional oligosaccharides for improving human health. *Adv Nutr*. 2011 May;2(3):284-9.

4. Muñoz Martín T, de la Hoz Caballer B, Marañón Lizana F et al. Selective allergy to sheep's and goat's milk proteins. *Allergol Immunopathol (Madr)*. 2004 Jan-Feb;32(1):39-42.

5. Carroccio A, Cavataio F, Iacono G. Cross-reactivity between milk proteins of different animals. *Clin Exp Allergy*. 1999 Aug;29(8):1014-6.

6. Turck D. Cow's milk and goat's milk. *World Rev Nutr Diet*. 2013; 108:56-62.

7. Maskatia ZK, Davis CM. Perinatal environmental influences on goat's and sheep's milk allergy without cow's milk allergy. *Ann Allergy Asthma Immunol*. 2013 Dec; 111(6):574-5.

8. Yang Y, Bu D, Zhao X, Sun P, Wang J, Zhou L. Proteomic analysis of cow, yak, buffalo, goat and camel milk whey proteins: quantitative differential expression patterns. *J Proteome Res*. 2013 Apr 5;12(4):1660-7.

9. Jirillo F, Magrone T. Anti-inflammatory and anti-allergic properties of donkey's and goat's milk. *Endocr Metab Immune Disord Drug Targets*. 2014 Mar;14(1):27-37.

CHAPTER 7

Does Breastfeeding Provide Health Benefits in Childhood and Beyond?

Experts recommend the exclusive use of breast milk for the first six months of life with gradual addition of foods thereafter as the child grows. Several lines of evidence indicate that benefits to the child accrue not only during the period of breastfeeding but also long-term, extending into adulthood. This is attributed to a variety of human milk components specific to humans.

For example, human milk contains nucleotides that are missing in cow's milk. These nucleotides play a critical role in digestive and immune systems as well as variety of metabolic processes.

Not just genetic transfection, these nucleotides contribute to creating a healthy bacterial balance in the baby's immature gut which in turn primes up the baby's undeveloped immune and metabolic systems for the rest of the life.

BENEFITS DURING BREASTFEEDING

HEALTHY DIGESTIVE SYSTEM

Mom's milk provides stimulatory and protective factors that help:

- Intestinal defenses including provision of antibodies and white blood cells that protect against infections and colitis

- Healthy growth of gut

- Improves healthy movement of gastrointestinal functions

- Against inflammation including colitis via the provision of anti-inflammatory components in milk

- Promotes the growth of beneficial bacteria in gut

As compared to use of formula milk, babies fed mother's milk show:

- Better emptying of stomach

- Greater levels of digestive enzymes especially in pre-term babies

- Reduced risk of necrotizing colitis

- Lower risk of diarrhea: In fact, formula-fed babies suffer twice as many diarrheal illnesses as compared to breast fed ones.

PREVENTION OF ILLNESS DURING BREASTFEEDING

- Lower incidence of fever after immunizations.

- Lower frequency of respiratory infections: The Howie study demonstrated that breastfed babies have 26.6% incidence of respiratory infections as compared to 37% among those who are fed a formula.

- Decreased rate of urinary tract infections (UTI): Dr. Pisacane and colleagues from the Università di Napoli, Italy, conducted a case control study of 128 infants with UTI and 128 infants admitted with any other acute illness. These investigators documented that breast feeding is protective against urinary tract infections.

- Goldblum and colleagues examined the secretion of defensive immune factors in urine and demonstrated that "the urinary excretion of all factors except lysozyme was 7- to 150-fold greater in infants fed human milk than in those fed cow's milk formula."

- Reduced incidence of ear infections: Dr. Dewey and colleagues from the University of California, Davis Medical Center found that breastfed babies suffered 19% fewer cases of otitis media. The results were even more pronounced (80% lower) when prolonged episodes of greater than 10 days were considered.

LONG TERM BENEFITS

Evidence suggests that beneficial effect of breastfeeding continue well past into adult life.

FEWER INFECTIONS AND CHRONIC ILLNESSES

Human whey proteins have generous amounts of lactoferrin, lysozyme, and human specific IgA antibodies that enhance baby's defenses. Cow's milk has little of these protective components.

Increasing amount of data comparing breastfeeding to formula feeding suggests that breastfeeding babies subsequently have:

- Fewer acute illnesses including fewer ear infections

- Lower rate of chronic illnesses

- Possible protection against obesity: Although some have characterized the association between breastfeeding and obesity as an "obesity-related myth", this concept has been challenged by many others who argue that the improved benefit, albeit small, is real and cannot be ignored.

- Reduced rate of hospitalizations

- Superior nervous system development

- Reduced severity of asthma as evidenced by fewer hospitalizations related to asthma

- Lower risk of pneumonia: Chantry and colleagues from the University of California, Davis Medical Center analyzed the National Health and Nutrition Examination Survey III, a nationally representative cross-sectional home survey conducted from 1988 to 1994. They demonstrated that babies who were breastfed for 4 to 6 months suffered 4-fold greater risk of pneumonia than those who were breastfed for greater than 6 months.

HOW CAN MILK AFFECT RISK FOR ALLERGIES

Human milk is rich in biologically active components including antibodies, growth factors, polyunsaturated fatty acids, and white blood cells that can impact immune system.

- Animal studies have shown that allergenic substances in the air and inhaled by lactating animal are then secreted in milk. This transfer through milk results in the stimulation of a specific tolerance to the allergan in the baby.

- Breast milk, while protective against infectious organisms, selectively supports growth of beneficial probiotic bacteria in the gut. This causes low "healthy" levels of infectious stimulation that induces a beneficial, controlled immune response instead of uncontrolled inflammation, thus helping build a healthy immune system for the long term.

The dynamic changes in milk components provide a healthy and age-appropriate immune system regulation in the baby. Breastfed babies absorb smaller amounts of food allergans as compared to formula-fed babies, likely as a result of a strengthened intestinal barrier.

The major human whey protein is lactalbumin. In contrast, cow's milk whey protein is mainly lactoglobulin, which may contribute to milk protein allergies as well as intestinal colic.

Breastfeeding may only be one of several factors involved in risk for future allergies. Hence the studies exclusively examining babies at high risk for allergies due to their genetic make-up are more likely to show any benefit. Studies that include children at average risk may require extremely large numbers of participants, in the absence of which, no significant advantage may be seen.

SKIN ECZEMA OR ATOPIC DERMATITIS

Exclusive breast feeding and use of hydrolyzed (semi-digested) formula reduces the risk of atopic dermatitis in children at high risk due to family history, etc.

Dr. Grulee and colleagues from Rush Medical College in Chicago, Illinois, studied a cohort of 20,061 babies for association of milk with infantile eczema and published their findings in the *Journal of Pediatrics*. They found the incidence of skin eczema in their infants to be the lowest among the breastfed babies. It was twice as high in those who were partially breastfed and as high as 7-fold among those fed formula milk.

Since the study by Dr. Grulee and colleagues documenting differences between effects of breast feeding and artificial feeding on atopic dermatitis in kids, there have been numerous studies yielding conflicting results.

A systematic review and meta-analysis by Dr. Gdalevich and colleagues concluded that exclusive breastfeeding for the first 3 months of life correlates with decreased incidence of atopic dermatitis. The beneficial effect is pronounced in kids with a family history of allergies.

They recommended that *"breastfeeding should be strongly recommended to mothers of infants with a family history of atopy"* as a strategy to prevent skin eczema in the child.

Similarly, Dr. Yang and colleagues from the Taipei Medical University Hospital performed a meta-analysis and demonstrated that exclusive breastfeeding as compared to formula milk is associated with a reduced risk of skin eczema or atopic dermatitis.

Strengthening the argument for milk consumption linked to eczema are the studies showing benefit of using hydrolyzed (semi-digested milk with broken down milk proteins) formula instead of cow's milk formula. Positive results from the use of hydrolyzed formulas can last as long as six years.

Some studies have shown a positive benefit from the use of partially hydrolyzed formulas even in kids with established atopic dermatitis resulting in fewer recurrences. Jin and colleagues studied 113 infants less than 6 months of age in a randomized controlled manner. Infants received partially hydrolyzed cow's milk formula or conventional cow's milk formula. The frequency and severity of episodes of atopic dermatitis was significantly reduced in the intervention group without any difference in growth rates.

Incidence of eczema is not just decreased by breastfeeding during infancy but is sustained over the long term. Dr. Kull and co-investigators reported that exclusive breast feeding for the first 4 months of life protects against eczema up to at least 4 years of age.

ASTHMA

Breastfed babies demonstrate lower risk of recurrent wheezing up to age 6 years.

Dr. Dogaru and colleagues performed a systematic review and meta-analysis of studies on breastfeeding and risk for asthma. Breastfeeding strongly protected against wheezing/asthma for the first two years although the positive effects waned over time.

OTHER CHRONIC CONDITIONS

HEALTHY STRONG BONES

Minerals in mother's milk are present in unique digestible complexes that allow them to be easily absorbed and available to the baby for bone health and metabolism.

Dr. Jones and colleagues from the Menzies Centre for Population Health Research, Tasmania, Australia, studied 330 eight-year old children. Breastfed kids had superior bone mineral density as compared to those fed formula milk. The investigators concluded that there is a healthy link between breastfeeding and subsequent bone mass in 8-year old children.

EYE HEALTH

Visual function is superior among kids fed human milk as compared to formula. According to Dr. Anderson and colleagues from the Oregon Health Sciences University, *"docosahexaenoic acid is the preferred dietary n-3 fatty acid for the development of the brain and retina."* As mentioned earlier, DHA is seen breast milk but not in cow's milk.

Incidence of retinopathy in pre-term babies is higher among formula fed as compared to breastfed premature babies. The Carlson study from the University of Tennessee, Memphis has shown that marine-oil-supplemented formula improves vision among pre-term infants up to 4 months of age by presumably by enhancing DHA levels available to the baby.

CANCER

Breastfed infants have a lower risk of lymphoma, leukemia, uterine and all childhood cancers. There are more details in succeeding chapters.

DIABETES MELLITUS

Breastfed infants may be less likely to develop type 1 as well as type 2 diabetes mellitus in later life. This issue is discussed in more detail in succeeding chapters.

HEART DISEASE

Although the studies are mixed, indirect data indicates that breastfed infants have a lower risk for adult cardiovascular disease. There are more details in succeeding chapters.

BRAIN HEALTH

I have devoted an entire chapter #9 to this topic. Chapter #10 discusses the topic of a possible link of cow milk consumption to autism.

Note: Babies breastfed for a prolonged period are at risk for iron deficiency anemia.

REFERENCES

1. Hauk L. AAFP Releases Position Paper on Breastfeeding. *Am Fam Physician*. 2015 Jan 1;91(1):56-7.

2. Pisacane A, Continisio P, Palma O et al. Breastfeeding and risk for fever after

immunization. *Pediatrics*. 2010 Jun;125(6):e1448-52.

3. Pisacane A, Graziano L, Mazzarella G, Scarpellino B, Zona G. Breast-feeding and urinary tract infection. *J Pediatr*. 1992 Jan;120(1):87-9.

4. Goldblum RM, Schanler RJ, Garza C et al. Human milk feeding enhances the urinary excretion of immunologic factors in low birth weight infants. *Pediatr Res*. 1989 Feb;25(2):184-8.

5. Dewey C, Midgeley E, Maw R. The relationship between otitis media with effusion and contact with other children in a british cohort studied from 8 months to 3 1/2 years. The ALSPAC Study Team. Avon Longitudinal Study of Pregnancy and Childhood. *Int J Pediatr Otorhinolaryngol*. 2000 Sep 15;55(1):33-45.

6. Chantry CJ, Howard CR, Auinger P. Full breastfeeding duration and associated decrease in respiratory tract infection in US children. *Pediatrics*. 2006 Feb;117(2):425-32.

7. Kramer MS, Kakuma R. Optimal duration of exclusive breastfeeding. *Cochrane Database Syst Rev.* 2012 Aug 15;8:CD003517.

8. Yamakawa M, Yorifuji T, Kato T et al. Long-Term Effects of Breastfeeding on Children's Hospitalization for Respiratory Tract Infections and Diarrhea in Early Childhood in Japan. *Matern Child Health J.* 2015 Feb 6.

9. Ajetunmobi OM, Whyte B, Chalmers J et al. and Glasgow Centre for Population Health Breastfeeding Project Steering Group. Breastfeeding is associated with reduced childhood hospitalization: evidence from a Scottish Birth Cohort (1997-2009). J Pediatr.2015 Mar;166(3):620-5.e4.

10. Yamakawa M, Yorifuji T, Inoue S, Kato T, Doi H. Breastfeeding and obesity among schoolchildren: a nationwide longitudinal survey in Japan. *JAMA Pediatr.*2013 Oct;167(10):919-25.

11. Yamakawa M, Yorifuji T, Kato T, Yamauchi Y, Doi H. Breast-feeding and hospitalization for asthma in early childhood: a nationwide longitudinal survey in Japan. *Public Health Nutr*. 2014 Nov 6:1-6.

12. Casazza K, Pate R, Allison DB. Myths, presumptions, and facts about obesity. N Engl J Med. 2013 Jun 6;368(23):2236-7.

13. Dogaru CM, Nyffenegger D, Pescatore AM, Spycher BD, Kuehni CE. Breastfeeding and childhood asthma: systematic review and meta-analysis. *Am J Epidemiol*. 2014 May 15;179(10):1153-67.

14. Yang YW, Tsai CL, Lu CY. Exclusive breastfeeding and incident atopic dermatitis in childhood: a systematic review and meta-analysis of prospective cohort studies. *Br J Dermatol*. 2009 Aug;161(2):373-83.

15. Jones G, Riley M, Dwyer T. Breastfeeding in early life and bone mass in prepubertal children: a longitudinal study. *Osteoporos Int*. 2000;11(2):146-52.

16. Howie PW. Protective effect of breastfeeding against infection in the first and second six months of life. *Adv Exp Med Biol*. 2002;503:141-7.

17. Pisacane A, Graziano L, Mazzarella G et al. Breast-feeding and urinary tract infection. J Pediatr. 1992 Jan;120(1):87-9.

18. Bode L. Human milk oligosaccharides: every baby needs a sugar mama. *Glycobiology*. 2012 Sep; 22(9):1147-62.

CHAPTER 8

Benefits for Breastfeeding Moms

HEALTH BENEFITS FOR THE MOM

Benefits accrue to the mom not just during the period of breastfeeding but far beyond. This is suggested by the fact that the beneficial effect of immune cells present in milk are not just seen in the baby but also in the lactating mammary gland.

IMMEDIATE HEALTH BENEFITS

- Recuperation from stress of childbirth is faster since breastfeeding stimulates oxytocin which in turn returns uterus to pre-delivery form.

- Lactating mothers suffer less stress. Lactation-induced hormonal changes have beneficial impact on social interactions including bonding with the baby. Breastfed babies are much less likely to suffer child abuse and neglect.

- Breastfeeding mothers have greater weight loss after delivery.

LONG-TERM MATERNAL BENEFITS

- Mothers with gestational diabetes have better glucose tolerance if they breastfeed the baby. Breastfeeding for over 3 months decreases the long term risk of diabetes type-2 in mothers with gestational diabetes.

- Breastfeeding reduces risk of breast and ovarian cancer.

- Some, but not all, studies indicate that breastfeeding mothers have stronger bone health.

- Multiple studies have documented the protective impact of breastfeeding against cardiovascular diseases.

- Breastfeeding lowers the risk of osteoporosis.

ECONOMIC BENEFITS FOR FAMILY AND SOCIETY

These may be assessed at both the family level as well as the society at large.

- Some experts argue that the value of human milk should be accounted for in gross national product. For example, the value of human milk accounts for $3 billion each year in Australia.

- A typical family directly saves about $1,000 per year in milk formula costs. The family does not need to worry about measuring formula and sterilizing the nipples etc, while saving money at the same time.

- Since breastfed babies suffer less sickness, it also results in savings from fewer doctor visits, reduced need for medications, fewer hospitalizations etc.

- Assuming over 80% babies are exclusively breastfed for at least 6 months, savings in US at national level have been estimated to be $13 billion.

REFERENCES

1. Gertosio C, Meazza C, Pagani S, Bozzola M. Breast feeding: gamut of benefits. *Minerva Pediatr*. 2015 May 29.

2. Chua S, Arulkumaran S, Lim I et al. Influence of breastfeeding and nipple stimulation on postpartum uterine activity. *Br J Obstet Gynaecol*. 1994 Sep;101(9):804-5.

3. Bode L, McGuire M, Rodriguez JM et al. It's alive: microbes and cells in human milk and their potential benefits to mother and infant. *Adv Nutr*. 2014 Sep;5(5):571-3.

4. Much D, Beyerlein A, Roßbauer M, Hummel S et al. Beneficial effects of breastfeeding in women with gestational diabetes mellitus. *Mol Metab*. 2014 Jan21;3(3):284-92.

5. González-Jiménez E, García PA, Aguilar MJ et al. Breastfeeding and the prevention of breast cancer: a retrospective review of clinical histories. *J Clin Nurs*. 2014 Sep;23(17-18):2397-403.

6. Smith JP. "Lost milk?": Counting the economic value of breast milk in gross domestic product. *J Hum Lact*. 2013 Nov;29(4):537-46.

Section III

Milk Matters

CHAPTER 9

Brain Health: Does Type of Milk Matter?

To argue with a person who has renounced the use of reason is like administering medicine to the dead.

---Thomas Paine

COMPOSITION OF MOM'S MILK IS DYNAMIC

The concentration of some but not all components in milk varies among women depending on the duration of breast feeding and even depending on time of the day. The composition may at times be different between right and left breast. This dynamic composition allows milk to meet the infant's requirements as needed. Overall, breast milk feeding is associated with superior brain development.

For example, human milk casein, when processed in the baby's gut, mimics a morphine-like substance called casomorphin that can affect the baby's mood and behavior. This early priming of behavior may have a life-long impact on the ultimate personality profile.

ABUNDANCE OF MEDICAL STUDIES TO LEARN FROM

DIFFERENCES IN BRAIN ELECTRICAL ACTIVITY

According to Dr. Jing and colleagues from the Arkansas Children's Nutrition Center, Little Rock, Arkansas, there are significant differences in the development of electrical activity in the brains of breastfed babies as compared to those fed cow milk or soy based formula. This illustrates that the type of diet/milk can affect brain development with potential for variations in future cognitive function among different people.

EFFECT ON SYLLABLE DISCRIMINATION

Studies by Dr. Pivik and colleagues have shown greater syllable discrimination in breastfed more than formula-fed babies.

EFFECT ON COGNITIVE AND PERFORMANCE TESTS

A recent study by Dr. Andres and colleagues from the Arkansas Children's Nutrition Center puts the spotlight on differences between human milk, cow's milk-based formula, and soy-based formula milk. While there was no difference between cow-based or soy-based milk formula consumers, the breastfed babies fared better on cognitive function and performance tests at six and twelve months of age.

BREASTFEEDING AND INTELLIGENCE

Several studies have reported superior intelligence and brain development in infants who are breastfed.

Mortensen and colleagues studied the correlation between duration of breast feeding and adult intelligence as a measure of brain development. Subjects were divided into 5 groups based on length of breastfeeding. Intelligence was estimated on the basis of the Wechsler Adult Intelligence Scale (WAIS) at age 27.2 years and the Børge Priens Prøve (BPP) test at age 18.7 years.

Results demonstrated that the longer the duration of breastfeeding, the higher the scores on the Verbal, Performance, and Full Scale WAIS IQs. The scores were as follows:

- Breastfeeding less than 1 month
  99.4

- Breastfeeding 2-3 months
  101.7

- Breastfeeding 4-6 months
  102.3

- Breastfeeding 7-9 months
  106.0

- Breastfeeding more than 9 months
  104.0

Scores on BPP tests also demonstrated superiority of breast milk:

- Breastfeeding less than 1 month
  38.0

- Breastfeeding 2-3 months
  39.2

- Breastfeeding 4-6 months
  39.9

- Breastfeeding 7-9 months
  40.1

- Breastfeeding more than 9 months
  40.1

The investigators concluded that after taking confounding factors into account, *"a significant positive association between duration of breastfeeding and intelligence was observed in 2 independent samples of young adults, assessed with 2 different intelligence tests."*

Similar to the above results, Kramer and colleagues found that Wechsler Abbreviated Scales of Intelligence measured at 6.5 years of age was superior among kids who had a more exclusive breastfeeding at 3 months of age and of any breastfeeding through one year of age as compared to the control subjects. The test scores increased by 7.5 for the verbal IQ and 2.9 for the performance IQ.

SUPERIORITY ON BRITISH ABILITY SCALES

Dr. Quigley and colleagues from the UK studied over 11,000 kids. These children were administered British Ability Scales tests of naming vocabulary, pattern construction, and picture similarities at age 5 years.

These investigators found that full-term breastfed children demonstrated a two-point increase in scores for picture similarities when breastfed for equal to or more than 4 months and naming vocabulary scores when breastfed equal to or more than 6 months.

In pre-term babies the advantage was even higher leading authors to conclude that *"breastfed children will be 1 to 6 months ahead of children who were never breastfed"*.

RECEPTIVE LANGUAGE, VERBAL AND NONVERBAL IQ

Belfort and colleagues from the Harvard Medical School performed a prospective cohort study to examine the correlations between breastfeeding and level of cognition at age 3 and 7 years. 1,312 subjects were included from Project Viva, a US pre-birth study group.

Receptive language was investigated at age 3 using the Peabody Picture Vocabulary Test. Wide Range Assessment of Visual Motor Abilities was performed at ages 3 and 7. Kaufman Brief Intelligence Test which looks at verbal and non-verbal intelligence and Wide Range Assessment of visual abilities, fine motor, memory and learning were administered at 7 years of age.

Results demonstrated that the duration of breastfeeding was directly proportional to superior receptive language development at 3 years and verbal as well as nonverbal IQ scores at school age.

EFFECT ON BEHAVIOR

Dr. Hekla and colleagues from the Finnish Institute of Occupational Health, in Helsinki, Finland analyzed data from the Millennium Cohort Study to examine links between breastfeeding and child behavior. 10,037 mother-child pairs were included in the analysis. Parents completed a behavior questionnaire. In addition, the Strengths and Difficulties Questionnaire was used for assessment.

These investigators documented that longer duration of breast feeding correlates with fewer behavioral issues in kids aged 5 years.

ANY RISKS TO BREASTFEEDING AS A POLICY?

A meta-analysis and systematic review conducted by Drs. Kramer and Kakuma concluded that there is no risk in *"in recommending, as a general policy, exclusive breastfeeding for the first six months of life in both developing and developed-country settings."*

BREASTFEEDING IS SUPERIOR, BUT CAN FORMULA MILK BE TOXIC?

Andres and colleagues compared the development status of 12-month babies fed mothers' milk as compared to cow's milk or a soy milk formula. Soya beans are rich in bioactive compounds and have the potential to affect development. Many infant formulas are soy-based.

The investigators demonstrated that breastfed babies had better Mental Developmental Index (MDI) scores as compared to soy-formula fed babies. The breastfed babies also had superior psycho-development as compared with those on a milk-based formula.

The study suggested a possible link between soy-based infant formula and more severe autistic behaviors in sub-domains of inappropriate speech among females, hypersensitivity to sensory stimulation in males and communication deficits among both males and females. Although a true cause-effect relationship remains to be established, it does suggest that soy milk may not always be a great substitute for breast milk.

HOW IS HUMAN MILK BENEFICIAL TO A CHILD'S BRAIN

The reports outlined above suggest that one or more components of breast milk may be critical for cognitive development. But what could be those beneficial components be?

BETTER METABOLIC AND ANTIOXIDANT FUNCTION

Human milk has higher levels of amino acid cysteine. Cysteine is critical for manufacture of glutathione, an antioxidant and for taurine that is required for not just metabolism in liver but also for healthy brain development.

LONG-CHAIN POLYUNSATURATED FATTY ACIDS IN HUMAN MILK HELP

According to Dr. Uauy and colleagues, essential fatty acids are contained in all tissues. However, the brain, retina and other nervous system components contain and require especially high amounts of these long-chain polyunsaturated fatty acids (LC-PUFA).

Human milk contains particularly generous amounts of very long-chain fatty acids like arachidonic acid and docosahexaenoic acid (DHA) that are synthesized from the essential fatty acids. These arachidonic and docosahexaenoic acids have been associated with improved brain development, cognition, growth, and vision.

DHA deficiency in animals has been shown to be harmful for neurobehavioral development. Manifestations include increased risk of anxiety, aggression, and depression. Likewise in humans, pre-term babies have lower levels of DHA in brain and are at a higher risk for neurobehavioral problems like attention-deficit hyperactivity disorder (ADHD) and schizophrenia

Dr. Uauy's laboratory has also shown that low levels of alpha-linolenic acid and docosahexaenoic acid (DHA) contribute to poorer functional development of the retina and parts of brain controlling vision.

DHA is not only critical to a functioning retina and the brain areas controlling vision, but also for development of the neurotransmitters required for transmission of electrochemical communication signals and overall functional maturation of the communication network in the central nervous system.

LOWER LEVELS OF LONG-CHAIN POLYUNSATURATED FATTY ACIDS IN FORMULA MILK

Formula milk has relatively higher amounts of medium chain-length fatty acids as compared to human milk. This supplementation of medium chain-length fatty acids results in relatively lower amounts of long-chain fatty acids in formula milk.

EFFECT OF SUPPLEMENTATION OF LONG-CHAIN POLYUNSATURATED FATTY ACIDS

The above notwithstanding, the Qawasmi meta-analysis of studies examining long-chain fatty acid supplementation of formula milk has not demonstrated any impact of early brain development. However, human studies on the effect of such supplementation on later cognition and brain development are lacking.

ROLE OF GENETICS AND EPIGENETICS

Genetics also plays a significant role in ultimate manifestations consistent with the gene-environment interaction concept. Dr. Caspi and colleagues from the King's College London, England, have demonstrated that breastfed children have superior IQs than children not fed breast milk. This effect is likely related to the fatty acids available in breast milk and not in cow's milk.

The linkage between breastfeeding and IQ is further complicated by interactions of a child's genes and environment. For example, genetic variants of genes like FADS2 which is involved in the regulation of fatty acid metabolism can modify the beneficial effects of human milk on IQ.

NEURODEGENERATIVE DISORDERS LIKE PARKINSON'S AND MULTIPLE SCLEROSIS

This topic is discussed in detail in *chapter #11*.

HOW CAN COW'S MILK BE HARMFUL TO BABY

Multiple lines of evidence indicate that cow's milk has the potential to be harmful, at least in a subset of patients. Milk may however not be the sole factor involved when problems do occur. The factors involved in creating a perfect storm include:

- Amount and duration of cow milk consumption including type of cows involved

- Loss of protective benefits from breastfeeding

- Genetic predisposition of the person

- Exposure to other potential toxins like gluten etc.

- Effect of other environmental factors that may turn certain genes off or on

Most of human milk is in the form of easily digestible whey protein. Casein protein forms a minority fraction. The opposite is true in the case of cow's milk.

Whey protein in humans contains lower amounts of potentially harmful amino acids like phenylalanine, tyrosine, and methionine. Babies raised on cow's milk have higher amounts of these amino acids. While important, these amino acids, when present in large amounts, can harm the developing brain.

References

1. Reardon S. Gut-brain link grabs neuroscientists. *Nature*. 2014 Nov 13;515(7526):175-7.

2. Mortensen EL, Michaelsen KF, Sanders SA, Reinisch JM: The association between duration of breastfeeding and adult intelligence. *JAMA*. 2002;287(18):2365.

3. Kramer MS, Aboud F, Mironova E, Vanilovich I et al. Promotion of Breastfeeding Intervention Trial (PROBIT) Study Group: Breastfeeding and child cognitive development: new evidence from a large randomized trial. *Arch Gen Psychiatry*. 2008;65(5):578.

4. Neville MC, Keller RP, Seacat J, Casey CE, Allen JC, Archer P: Studies on human lactation. I. Within-feed and between-breast variation in selected components of human milk. *Am J Clin Nutr*. 1984;40(3):635.

5. Uauy R, Peirano P, Hoffman D, Mena P, Birch D, Birch E. Role of essential fatty acids in the function of the developing

nervous system. *Lipids*. 1996 Mar;31Suppl:S167-76.

6. Uauy R, Hoffman DR, Peirano P, Birch DG, Birch EE. Essential fatty acids in visual and brain development. *Lipids*. 2001 Sep;36(9):885-95.

7. Qawasmi A, Landeros-Weisenberger A, Leckman JF, Bloch MH. Meta-analysis of long-chain polyunsaturated fatty acid supplementation of formula and infant cognition. *Pediatrics*. 2012 Jun;129(6):1141-9.

8. Auestad N, Scott DT, Janowsky JS, Jacobsen C et al. Visual, cognitive, and language assessments at 39 months: a follow-up study of children fed formulas containing long-chain polyunsaturated fatty acids to 1 year of age. *Pediatrics*. 2003 Sep;112(3 Pt 1):e177-83.

9. McNamara RK, Carlson SE. Role of omega-3 fatty acids in brain development and function: potential implications for the pathogenesis and prevention of psychopathology. *Prostaglandins Leukot*

Essent Fatty Acids. 2006 Oct-Nov;75(4-5):329-49.

10. Quigley MA, Hockley C, Carson C, Kelly Y, Renfrew MJ, Sacker A: Breastfeeding is associated with improved child cognitive development: a population-based cohort study. *J Pediatr*. 2012;160(1):25.

11. Belfort MB, Rifas-Shiman SL, Kleinman KP, Guthrie LB, Bellinger DC, Taveras EM, Gillman MW, Oken E. Infant feeding and childhood cognition at ages 3 and 7 years: Effects of breastfeeding duration and exclusivity. *JAMA Pediatr*. 2013 Sep;167(9):836-44.

12. Caspi A, Williams B, Kim-Cohen J, Craig IW, Milne BJ, Poulton R, Schalkwyk LC, Taylor A, Werts H, Moffitt TE. Moderation of breastfeeding effects on the IQ by genetic variation in fatty acid metabolism. *Proc Natl Acad Sci U S A*. 2007 Nov 20;104(47):18860-5.

13. Heikkilä K, Sacker A, Kelly Y, Renfrew MJ, Quigley MA. Breast feeding and child behaviour in the Millennium Cohort

Study. *Arch Dis Child*. 2011 Jul;96(7):635-42.

14. Jing H, Gilchrist JM, Badger TM, Pivik RT. A longitudinal study of differences in electroencephalographic activity among breastfed, milk formula-fed, and soy formula-fed infants during the first year of life. *Early Hum Dev*. 2010 Feb;86(2):119-25.

15. Pivik RT, Andres A, Badger TM. Diet and gender influences on processing and discrimination of speech sounds in 3- and 6-month-old infants: a developmental ERP study. *Dev Sci*. 2011 Jul;14(4):700-12.

16. Andres A, Cleves MA, Bellando JB, Pivik RT, Casey PH, Badger TM. Developmental status of 1-year-old infants fed breast milk, cow's milk formula, or soy formula. *Pediatrics*. 2012 Jun;129(6):1134-40.

CHAPTER 10

Autism and Cow's Milk

I think that autistic brains tend to be specialized brains. Autistic people tend to be less social. It takes a ton of processor space in the brain to have all the social circuits.

---*Temple Grandin*

The opioid excess theory suggests that autism is a neuro-metabolic malfunction. Large amounts of biologically-active morphine-like opioid compounds from the breakdown of gluten and casein are absorbed through the leaky gut and enter the brain. They bind to the opioid binding sites in different regions of the brain to affect brain function.

Such a situation may occur in subjects who drink cow's milk but also have leaky gut with defective or deficient digestive enzymes. Continued consumption of cow's milk in such cases allows metabolically bio-active chemicals to enter the brain in toxic amounts.

Absorption of toxic compounds is likely to be higher during early formative years of life when the intestinal barrier is not mature. This fact alone has the potential to contribute to an increased harmful effect on the brain during its critical period of development.

WHAT DOES THE MEDICAL EVIDENCE SUGGEST?

ROLE OF CASOMORPHINS

Children with autism have higher levels of cow's casomorphin-7 immunoreactivity in the urine. Kaminski and colleagues have demonstrated that breakdown of cow's beta-casein variants results in variable amounts of bioactive peptide beta-casomorphin7 depending on the herd and breed. Very high levels of this potentially toxic biochemical are seen when the source of milk is from Holstein types of cattle breeds as compared to others. Holstein is the source of most milk in the west especially the U.S.

It is worth noting that neuro-behavioral disorders such as autism and schizophrenia seem to be associated with higher level of beta-casomorphin7.

Studies authored by Dr. Kost and colleagues from the National Research Center for Mental Health in Moscow, Russia, *"support the hypothesis for deterioration of bovine casomorphin elimination as a risk factor for delay in psychomotor development and other diseases such as autism."*

BREAKDOWN PRODUCTS OF COW'S MILK ARE DIFFERENT

Variability in peptides (smaller protein breakdown products) from human and cow's milk have been implicated in the neuro-developmental differences. Food-derived opioid peptides from wheat or milk cause reduced antioxidant capacity. This in turn may increase the risk of inflammation including low grade inflammation in the brains of genetically vulnerable children. This may explain the beneficial effect of a dietary exclusion of wheat and milk in some studies.

IS IT IATROGENIC AUTISM?

Rising incidence of autism has prompted Dr. Hahr from the Children's Hospital in Milwauki, WI to promote the term *"iatrogenic autism"*. He blames it on increasing use of formula milk for feeding babies. Most of the formula milk is cow based.

Dr. Hahr hypothesizes that because of the higher molecular weight of cow's milk as compared to human milk, there is altered hemo-dynamics in baby's circulation. This in turn results in abnormalities of blood-tissue-brain interactions.

HUMAN TRIALS

There is a paucity of peer-reviewed studies on the use of milk/casein exclusion from the diet of patients with neurobehavioral dysfunction. Many of them have been carried out in conjunction with a gluten-free diet and have shown positive impacts on certain autistic symptoms.

Dr. Lucarelli and colleagues studied the effect of diet in autism. They found that the patients with autism had higher levels of antibodies directed against milk protein casein as compared to healthy subjects.

These investigators further studied 36 patients with autism and treated them with a cow's milk casein exclusion diet along with an elimination of any foods for which subjects had positive skin test. The authors found a significant improvement in neurobehavioral function at 8 weeks. The symptoms worsened on the reintroduction of milk casein in their diet.

The *ScanBrit trial* that examined the effect of gluten-free casein-free diet also found a positive response in kids with autism.

IS A SOY-BASED FORMULA ALWAYS SAFE?

Soya beans are rich in bioactive compounds and have the potential to affect development. Many infant formulas are soy-based. One study showed a link between consumption of a soy-based infant formula and more severe autistic behaviors such as inappropriate speech among females, hypersensitivity to sensory stimulation in males and communication deficits among both males and females.

Studies done by Dr. Westmark from the Department of Neurology at the University of Wisconsin Medical Sciences Center, have demonstrated that soy-based infant formulae may be associated with autistic behaviors as well.

Dr. Westmark's studies have also shown that *"the use of soy-based infant formula may be associated with febrile seizures in both genders and with a diagnosis of epilepsy in males in autistic children."*

IS CAMEL MILK
BETTER OR WORSE FOR AUTISM?

Anecdotal evidence comes from case reports. For example, Dr. Adams reported that his son with autism experienced significant improvement once he started drinking one half cup of camel milk every day. This beneficial effect was sustained for 6 years.

One of the reasons might be that the camel milk does not contain certain allergens that are present in cow's milk, e.g. â-lactoglobulin and a "new" â-casein.

Thymus and activation-regulated chemokine (TARC) is a pro-inflammatory chemical that is increased in many kids with autism. Bashir and Al-Ayadhi conducted a double-blind, randomized, controlled trial for 2 weeks to examine the effect of camel milk, both raw and boiled, on the TARC levels as well as on the Childhood Autism Rating Scale in kids with autism.

Administration of camel milk, both raw and boiled, resulted in a reduction in TARC levels as compared to placebo. This was associated with a significant improvement in the clinical measurements of the score on Childhood Autism Rating Scale.

In contrast to antibodies from most mammals, camel IgG antibodies are comprised of heavy-chain antibodies and are devoid of a light chain. As such, the camel antibodies are much smaller and classified as nano-antibodies. Their size is about 1/10th the size of human antibodies. The small size allows them to be passed from the milk across the gut barrier and into the human circulation resulting in potential to modulate the immune balance in the entire human body including the brain.

BOTTOM-LINE ON THE LITERATURE

All milk is not the same. All casein proteins from different animals are not the same. With so much variability in the structural and functional components of milk from different sources, it is entirely possible that a combined casein-free and gluten-free diet as well other purported toxic dietary components have additive or even symbiotic beneficial impacts on behavior.

To be sure, negative studies of dietary interventions including gluten-free and casein-free diet have also been reported. Many of these have been short-term studies even though evidence suggests that at least a six month trial is needed to see a significant impact. An example is the study by Dr. Navarro and colleagues whose trial lasted one month and, by the authors' own admission, was too underpowered to detect a significant difference.

Since the data are somewhat inconsistent, an evolving view is that there is a sub-set of autism patients whose manifestations are mechanistically and therapeutically linked at least in part to diet.

It is noteworthy that a recent Israeli government report of social services documented a 500 % increase of autism in Israel between 2004 and 2011 and the speculation is that it is related to diet. The absolute numbers are quite low, however, compared to the West. This reported increase may also in part be related to awareness of autism, the stigma of autism diagnosis, and differences in health delivery programs.

REFERENCES

1. Mayer EA, Padua D, Tillisch K. Altered brain-gut axis in autism: comorbidity or causative mechanisms? Bioessays. 2014 Oct;36(10):933-9.

2. Schmidt C. Mental health: thinking from the gut. Nature. 2015 Feb 26;518(7540):S12-5.

3. Rosenfeld CS. Microbiome Disturbances and Autism Spectrum Disorders. Drug Metab Dispos. 2015 Apr 7.

4. Trivedi MS, Shah JS, Al-Mughairy S, Hodgson NW et al. Food-derived opioid peptides inhibit cysteine uptake with redox and epigenetic consequences. J Nutr Biochem. 2014 Oct;25(10):1011-8.

5. Sokolov O, Kost N, Andreeva O, Korneeva E, Meshavkin V et al. Autistic children display elevated urine levels of bovine casomorphin-7 immunoreactivity. Peptides.2014 Jun;56:68-71.

6. Lucarelli S., Frediani T., Zingoni A. M., Ferruzzi F., Giardini O., Quintieri F., et al. (1995). Food allergy and infantile autism. Panminerva Med. 37, 137–141.

7. Westmark CJ. Soy Infant Formula may be Associated with Autistic Behaviors. Autism Open Access. 2013 Nov 18;3

8. Westmark CJ. Soy infant formula and seizures in children with autism: a retrospective study. PLoS One. 2014 Mar 12;9(3):e80488.

9. Navarro F, Pearson DA, Fatheree N, Mansour R, Hashmi SS, Rhoads JM. Are 'leakygut' and behavior associated with gluten and dairy containing diet in children with autism spectrum disorders? Nutr Neurosci. 2015 May;18(4):177-85.

10. Reardon S. Gut-brain link grabs neuroscientists. Nature. 2014 Nov 13;515(7526):175-7.

11. Bashir S, Al-Ayadhi LY. Effect of camel milk on thymus and activation-regulated chemokine in autistic children: double-blind study. Pediatr Res. 2014 Apr;75(4):559-63.

12. Kost NV, Sokolov OY, Kurasova OB et al. Beta-casomorphins-7 in infants on different type of feeding and different levels of psychomotor development. Peptides. 2009 Oct;30(10):1854-60.

13. Marcason W. What is the current status of research concerning use of a gluten-free, casein-free diet for children diagnosed with autism? J Am Diet Assoc. 2009 Mar; 109(3):572.

14. Hsu CL, Lin CY, Chen CL, Wang CM et a. The effects of a gluten and casein-free diet in children with autism: a case report. Chang Gung Med J. 2009 Jul-Aug; 32(4):459-65.

15. Reichelt KL, Knivsberg AM. The possibility and probability of a gut-to-brain connection in autism. Ann Clin Psychiatry. 2009 Oct-Dec; 21(4):205-11.

16. Adams CM. Patient report: autism spectrum disorder treated with camel milk. Glob Adv Health Med. 2013 Nov;2(6):78-80.

17. Al-Ayadhi LY, Elamin NE. Camel Milk as a Potential Therapy as an Antioxidant in Autism Spectrum Disorder (ASD). Evid Based Complement Alternat Med. 2013;2013:602834.

CHAPTER 11

Diseases Linked to the Use of Cow's Milk

Medicine is not a science; it is an empiricism founded on a network of blunders.

---Emmet Densmore

INFANTILE COLIC

Babies fed cow's milk tend to have more problems with infantile colic. Children get relief from the colicky pain when they are fed pre-digested cow's milk. This suggests that either the complexity of cow's milk and/or the deficiency of digestive processes in the baby play a role in the pathogenesis of colic.

Dr. Lucassen from the Radbound University Nijmegen in The Netherlands, conducted a systematic review of effective remedies for infantile colic. They concluded that switching from cow's milk formula to a predigested protein-based or soy-based formula reduces infantile colic.

Another systematic review of 19 studies by Hall and colleagues from the Monash University in Victoria, Australia reached a similar conclusion stating that *"there is some scientific evidence to support the use of a casein hydrolysate (pre-digested) formula in formula-fed infants or a low-allergen maternal diet in breastfed infants with infantile colic."*

IRON DEFICIENCY ANEMIA

Multiple studies have documented that the early introduction of cow's milk, unless adequately supplemented, increases the risk of iron deficiency anemia in the baby. The factors include:

- Iron levels in cow's milk are low.

- Cow's milk has high concentrations of calcium as well as casein proteins. Both block the absorption of iron from the baby's gut.

- Occult (invisible to naked eye) blood loss from the gut occurs in as many as 40% of the babies fed cow's milk resulting in anemia.

OCCULT BLOOD LOSS IN COW-MILK FED BABIES

The cause such GI blood loss remains to be established.

The blood loss from the gut declines after the age of 1 year. Earlier recommendations included avoidance of cow's milk during at least in the first 12 months of life. They were later modified stating that a family's tradition and practices need to be considered in the decision and while small amounts of cow's milk may be consumed early on, it should not be the main source of nutrition.

"*Growing up milks*" are available on the market. These contain lower levels of proteins along with adequate mineral supplementation. The overall benefit of such commercial milk continues to be a matter of debate.

RISK FOR ALLERGIES

Human milk is less likely to cause allergic reactions in the baby, as it lacks many of the foreign proteins present in cow's milk. For example, milk from all different animals contain alpha-lactalbumin but the structure is different in different species. It is not surprising that human babies tolerate human lactalbumin the best.

Allergy to milk is common among patients with atopic dermatitis, next only to egg allergy. Dietary restrictions are helpful however only in patients with food allergies.

COW'S MILK ALLERGY

Cow's milk allergy is a well-known, widely prevalent, and growing problem in the West. It occurs in about 2 to 5 % of kids. Allergic reaction is usually due to milk's casein and/or whey proteins. It should be noted that some of the cow's milk allergens like bovine alpha-1 casein may also be found in human milk, but usually do not cause problems. Treatment involves complete exclusion of milk from diet. Sensitivity to cow's milk may also occur without the involvement of allergy mechanisms.

Switching the animal source of milk may help.

Some, but not all, kids who are allergic to cow's milk may be able to drink goat's milk. Camel's milk however has less cross-sensitivity with cow's milk and may be a better alternative than goat's milk for children with a cow's milk allergy.

Studies by Dr. Monti's laboratory indicate that donkey milk is well-tolerated by children with a cow's milk allergy.

Current evidence suggests that modification of intestinal bacteria using pre- and probiotics may be a possible therapeutic target for kids with a cow's milk allergy.

ACNE

Studies suggest that insulin-like growth factor may play a role in causation of acne. According to Dr. Melnik from the University of Osnabrück,

Germany, the *"rising incidence of acne in the Western society may be related to increased insulin- and IGF-1-stimulation of sebaceous glands mediated by milk consumption."* Hormonal changes induced by cow's milk causes changes in sebaceous glands leading to acne.

Many patients believe that a dietary trigger is responsible for their acne. Multiple studies have documented an association between cow's milk and acne. Adebamowo and colleagues analyzed the data from 47,355 women enrolled in Nurses Health Study II. They found a positive correlation between total as well as skimmed milk intake during high school and acne. These results were confirmed in multiple other studies including a prospective study done by same authors in 4,273 teenage boys.

Further case controlled and cross-sectional studies have further bolstered the argument that frequent milk consumption is linked to acne.

A case series of 5 patients demonstrated that whey protein precipitated flare up of acne in teenagers using whey protein for muscle building and increasing weight. 20% of cow's milk protein is comprised of whey which stimulates insulin secretion and is believed to be responsible for acne. Acne cleared in these teenagers upon discontinuation of whey supplementation.

LACTOSE INTOLERANCE: LACTASE DEFICIENCY OR LACTOSE SENSITIVITY?

Milk contains a large amount of lactose. The entity of lactose intolerance is not new. It was recognized as far back as Hippocrates. However, the clinical syndrome of lactose intolerance has only been appreciated in recent decades.

EFFECTS OF LACTASE DEFICIENCY

The clinical symptoms vary and the complex includes abdominal pain, bloating, diarrhea, gas. Upper GI symptoms such as nausea and vomiting may also occur. The metabolic products of undigested lactose include short chain fatty acids as well as increased intestinal gases of methane, carbon dioxide type. These gases can actually make the gut slow thus sometimes actually causing constipation.

The frequency and severity of symptoms varies based on the levels of lactase enzyme in the person and the foods concurrently consumed.

Patients with lactase deficiency can safely consume up to 11g of lactose per day without suffering side-effects. The threshold may be higher when consumed with certain foods and in small multiple portions. On the other hand, those prone to colic or IBS may suffer symptoms at much lower doses and may not even be able to tolerate 6g/day of lactose.

CAN SERIOUS SIDE EFFECTS OCCUR?

While rare, persistent consumption of high amounts of lactose in a lactase deficient person may give rise to high levels of galactitol as a breakdown product that can even cause blindness.

IS IT MILK ALLERGY?

Lactose intolerance is not the same as milk allergy. Most patients with lactose intolerance can tolerate about a glass of milk per day, especially when taken with a meal. Fermented milk is better tolerated since it contains less lactose.

It should be noted that most of us digest lactose very well in early childhood, and the ability declines as we grow older.

PERHAPS MOTHER NATURE IS TRYING TO TIP US OFF!

The cause of lactose intolerance is deficiency of the lactase enzyme, which breaks down the lactose in milk. The prevalence of lactose intolerance is high worldwide, depending upon race and ethnicity. It reaches as high as 90 % in some ethnic populations. The prevalence is low in Caucasians of Northern European descent and very high in Hispanics and African-Americans.

No wonder there has been an explosion of lactose-free products in the grocery stores.

Lactose intolerance is not as simple as it sounds. Controlled studies have actually shown that the severity of symptoms is not related to the severity of lactase deficiency.

Many patients continue to have symptoms after switching to a lactose-free diet, suggesting other factors may be at play. Could it be a *"milk sensitivity"* that is causing the GI symptoms?

Studies by Dr. Olivier and co-investigators indicate that sensitization to cow's milk, as manifested by increased antibodies to cow's milk proteins, may be involved.

EFFECT OF MILK ON GROWTH AND OTHER LONG-TERM CONSEQUENCES

According to Dr. Mølgaard and colleagues from the Department of Human Nutrition, University of Copenhagen, milk stimulates linear growth during childhood via its effect on hormones and the immune system. Its effect on insulin-like growth factor and insulin may have positive or negative long-term consequences.

Dr. Thorsdottir and colleagues reviewed effects of the consumption of cow's milk in early infancy and deemed it as having *"unfortunate effects on growth, especially weight acceleration and development of overweight in childhood."*

DIABETES MELLITUS TYPE 1

The incidence of type 1 DM has been rising in recent decades. The cause of the increase remains unknown.

SINGLE CAUSE OR MULTIPLE FACTORS

With so many competing and credible theories, it is likely that multiple factors and not just a single factor is involved. There may be a significant overlap of factors in different parts of the world depending on genetic makeup and the peculiarities of environment in that region.

ROLE OF IMMUNE FACTORS

Gut-associated immune tissue may play a critical role in autoimmune diseases. Animal studies in diabetes-prone rats have demonstrated that administration of cow's milk at an early stage not only increases the incidence but also the early onset of diabetes. The disease is also accelerated in the presence of cow's milk.

The immunological mechanisms are still unclear and there seems to be some overlap between the various factors.

THE MILK EFFECT

There are substantial differences in milk proteins derived from different types of cows depending on breed and how they are raised etc. There is potential for variable effects due to the different biological activities of different biologically-active proteins.

DIFFERENT RESULTS FROM DIFFERENT META-ANALYSIS

The Griebler meta-analysis found seven studies examining role of cow's milk and type 1 diabetes. The authors reported that 6 out of 7 studies did not find any significant effect.

A meta-analysis by Patelarou and colleagues yielded 161 studies. 28 of the 161 met inclusion criteria. Eight studies reported that breastfeeding reduces risk of type 1 diabetes development. Seven more studies found that a short period or lack of breastfeeding could increase risk for type 1 diabetes. Overall, the investigators concluded that *"a short duration and/or a lack of breastfeeding may constitute a risk factor for the development of T1D later in life."*

EFFECT OF HYDROLYZED COW'S MILK

Knip and colleagues conducted a double-blind, randomized trial of infants at high risk for developing future diabetes based on genetic makeup. They were administered a hydrolyzed (semi-digested) casein formula or a conventional, cow's-milk-based formula (control) during the first 6 to 8 months of life. There was an increased development of auto-antibodies against pancreas indicating that infants develop early beta-cell immunity related to development of diabetes.

HOW MAY COW'S MILK CAUSE DM1

There appears to be similarity or cross-reactivity between antibodies against cow's milk proteins and the antibodies against pancreas. Such antibodies can thus damage the pancreas and cause diabetes.

Not all components of cow's proteins are diabetogenic. Some of them interact with the human intestinal immune system triggering an immune reaction leading to the disease. For example, diabetogenic mice develop diabetes when given *b-casein A1*, but not of *b-casein A2*.

However, jury is still out on the effect of A1/A2 caseins on health in humans.

In recent years, as breastfeeding has declined, the use of formula has increased. It may be the combination of decline of protective breastfeeding and consumption of "harmful" cow's milk that may ultimately determine the fate of child health.

Early exposure to cow's milk coupled with high milk intake during childhood has been linked to the development of type 1 DM. The albumin and/or beta-casein in cow's milk have been implicated. However, data is contradictory and the jury is out on this issue.

Overall, it appears that starting cow's milk formula at an early age may have a detrimental impact on the intestine including increased inflammation, and hyper-permeability or leaky gut. This increases the potential for immune reaction to cow's milk proteins which can in turn interrupt and disrupt the healthy immune balance. As stated above, cow's milk as a culprit would be in conjunction with other factors and not the sole cause.

DIABETES MELLITUS TYPE 2 AND OBESITY?

BODY GETS PRIMED IN EARLY CHILDHOOD

Metabolic programming occurs during infancy. Early childhood dynamics along with environmental and nutritional factors can have a life-altering impact during this critical period of development.

We do know that a lack of breastfeeding is considered to be an important modifiable risk factor against development of both type 1 and 2 diabetes. It is unclear if the non-breastfed babies have greater risk due to substitution with cow's milk formula itself or because of a lack of specific protective factors that are normally present in human milk. The linkage of actual use of cow's milk thus can be termed as cloudy at best.

For example, some milk products like cheese and fermented dairy products actually have a favorable impact on glucose regulation in the body.

Gao and colleagues conducted a meta-analysis of 14 cohort studies and concluded that a *"a modest increase in daily intake of dairy products such as low fat dairy, cheese and yogurt"* may result in lower risk for type 2 diabetes.

Likewise, Chen and colleagues found that increased consumption of yogurt is associated with a decreased risk of type 2 diabetes; other dairy products do not have any significant impact.

It should be noted that fermented milk products do not have the same properties as regular milk. Fermented products have healthy probiotic bacteria that have beneficial effects on gut and immune system. Probiotics have been shown to be of benefit in diabetes.

CARDIOVASCULAR HEALTH

Just like any other food, milk contains components that can help, as well as components that can harm. The overall protective or detrimental effect depends on the sum total of these components. It is not surprising that different studies have come up with different results.

The high fat and cholesterol content of milk has been pointed out as possibly causing higher risk for cardiovascular disease. For example, palmitic acid in milk increases bad fats, and myristic increases cholesterol. In contrast however, lauric acid increases good fat thus resulting in a protective function.

DO WE HAVE CONCLUSIVE PROOF?

While overall there does not appear to be a conclusive proof that milk is detrimental to heart health, Dr. Hu and colleagues have shown that higher ratio of high-fat to low-fat dairy consumption was linked to higher risk of cardiovascular risk among women.

Studies by Dr. Larsson and colleagues demonstrated that while milk consumption is not linked to stroke, whole milk is associated with an increased risk for intra-cerebral hemorrhage. In a similar study carried out in a different population, Larsson's group demonstrated that low fat dairy actually is inversely related to stroke.

Based on the data outlined above, it would be unfair to assume that whole milk is risk-free in subjects otherwise prone to heart disease, for example subjects with diabetes.

PROTECTIVE MILK COMPONENTS

Some of the bio-active components of milk can help lower blood pressure. Hypertension is a risk factor for heart disease and stroke. The beneficial effects of milk consumption include low fat milk lowering blood pressure in patients with hypertension.

SOME STUDIES SHOW PROTECTIVE OR NO EFFECT

Kondo and colleagues have shown that the use of milk and other dairy products is inversely linked to cardiovascular death.

On the other hand, the *Rotterdam study* with Dr. Praagman as the lead author demonstrated that total dairy consumption or the ingestion of any specific dairy products is not related to a risk of cardiovascular disease.

PARKINSON'S DISEASE

It is a neurodegenerative disorder and the cause remains to be established. Evidence points to environmental factors like pollution, pesticides, toxins etc. on top of genetic susceptibility. Leaky gut has been implicated since the gut may act as one of the major ports of entry of toxins into the body.

Multiple studies from the US and Europe have shown a positive link between milk consumption and Parkinson's disease.

Jiang and colleagues from the Qingdao University Medical College in the People's Republic of China conducted a meta-analysis of prospective cohort studies to determine the correlation between dairy food consumption and risk of Parkinson's disease. Seven studies with 1,083 cases of Parkinson's among 304,193 subjects were included in the data analysis. Results showed that the combined risk of Parkinson's for the highest as compared to lowest level of dairy foods intake was 1.40 overall, with the risk being higher for men (1.66) than women (1.15) for women.

Overall, the risk appears to be stronger for milk as compared to cheese, butter, yogurt etc. Which of the milk components are responsible for harm remains to be established. The fact that leaky gut has been implicated as playing a role in allowing the entry of potential toxins into the gut and the fact that lactase deficiency is common resulting in mal-digestion of milk suggests that the correlation is not merely due to an association but there may be a causative element.

In the absence of evidence to the contrary, skeptics like Kistner and Krack from the University Hospital Grenoble in France maintain that that the link between milk and Parkinson's is merely an association and does not reflect a cause-effect relationship. The jury is still out on this issue.

MULTIPLE SCLEROSIS

Ingestion of cow milk has been implicated in pathogenesis of neuro-degenerative disorders like multiple sclerosis. A cow milk factor, if involved, has not yet been identified.

Dr. Whitley and colleagues from Germany studied the following:

- Blood from healthy cattle

- Commercial milk available on the market

- Blood and brain tissue from patients with multiple sclerosis

DNA was extracted from milk, blood and tissues and compared.

The commercial cow's milk, healthy cattle blood as well as blood and tissues from patients with MS demonstrated 11 distinct DNA molecules similar to those seen in another brain disorder called *transmissible spongiform encephalopathy*.

Does this mean cow's milk is involved in multiple sclerosis? Hardly. But the tantalizing results of the study suggest that it sure is biologically plausible.

CANCER

The terms cancer and food are not monolithic. Carcinogenesis itself is a complex process. Adding to the complexity are different types of cancers in different types of organs. The relationship with food is complicated not just by different types of foods and dietary patterns but also by the presence of protective and carcinogenic factors in the same food product.

As a measure of a dietary component, dairy products are a heterogeneous group of foods and their make-up varies by region. It is not easy to attribute an effect to a single food or food product in its original form or after it has been developed into another product.

No wonder, data from various studies, both experimental and human subjects, points in different directions.

POTENTIALLY CANCER-CAUSING COMPONENTS IN MILK

The harmful effects of milk in cancer are largely attributed to its fat content and the insulin-like growth factor (IGF-1).

Several cross sectional studies and randomized controlled trials as well as meta-analysis have shown that milk intake increases IGF-1 in blood which in turn has been associated with higher risk of cancers of the breast and prostate.

Excessive fat consumption can affect male and female hormones in the body, altering their healthy balance and thus have the potential to affect a risk of breast and prostate cancers.

INCONTROVERTIBLE FACT ABOUT BOVINE GROWTH HORMONE

Recombinant bovine growth hormone (rBGH) increases cow's milk production by as much as 15 %. The use of rBGH for enhancing cow milk production is allowed in the U.S. In contrast, this practice is banned in the European Union.

Cows given rBGH have increased concentrations of insulin-like growth factor (IGF-1). According to the American Cancer Society, while there may be a link between high IGF-1 blood levels and cancer, the exact nature of this link remains unclear.

EFFECT OF LACTOSE INTOLERANCE

Galactose derived from lactose has toxic effects in the body, especially in ovaries. High levels of galactose are seen in patients with a lactase deficiency. As can be expected, individuals with lactose intolerance tend to avoid milk. Ji and colleagues from the Lund University of Sweden studied the link between lactose intolerance and cancer risk. A total of 22,788 subjects were included. The subjects with lower dairy intake had a lower risk of lung, breast and ovarian cancers.

DIGESTIVE CANCERS

European Prospective Investigation into Cancer and Nutrition (EPIC) study examined the relationship between colorectal cancer and milk products (whole-fat, semi-skimmed and skimmed). The study involved 477,122 men and women. The authors led by Dr. Murphy from the Imperial College London, London, United Kingdom concluded that dairy products have a protective effect against colorectal cancer.

On the other hand, an ecologic study by Abbastabar and colleagues found that dairy consumption is a risk factor for colorectal cancer.

Available evidence also indicates that dairy consumption is not a risk factor for gastric cancer or pancreatic cancer.

PROSTATE CANCER

Aune and colleagues from the Norwegian University of Science and Technology, Trondheim, Norway, conducted a meta-analysis of possible links between dairy and prostate cancer. 32 studies were included. The investigators found that increasing consumption of milk, low-fat milk, and cheese tend to prostate cancer risk.

OVARIAN CANCER

The relationship with ovarian cancer remains controversial since different meta-analysis of studies have come to conflicting conclusions.

BLADDER CANCER

Dairy intake reduces risk for bladder cancer.

BREAST CANCER

Dong and colleagues conducted a meta-analysis of prospective cohort studies to examine risk of dairy consumption and breast cancer. 18 studies involving 24,187 cases and 1,063,471 participants met the inclusion criteria. Results showed that higher intake of total dairy products and not just milk may be associated with a decreased risk of breast cancer.

A CONTRARIAN VIEW POINT

Above notwithstanding, some studies do in fact show adverse impact of milk consumption in high quantities.

WORLD CANCER RESEARCH FUND SUMS IT UP

The World Cancer Research Fund and American Institute for Cancer Research treatise on the association of food, nutrition, physical activity, and the prevention of cancer concluded that "*the evidence on the relationship between milk and dairy products, and also diets high in calcium, and the risk of cancer, points in different directions. Milk probably protects against colorectal cancer. Diets high in calcium are a probable cause of prostate cancer; there is limited evidence suggesting that high consumption of milk and dairy products is a cause of prostate cancer*".

IS THERE A POSSIBILITY OF DELAY IN RECOGNITION OF HARMFUL EFFECTS: THE GLUTEN AND IBS ANALOGY

For many years, patients were claiming that their symptoms of irritable bowel syndrome (IBS) would get better upon excluding gluten from their diet. However, the medical community frequently poked fun at that notion, since these patients did fulfill the criteria for diagnosis of celiac disease. We know now from clinical studies that many of the patients with IBS have what we now call "non-celiac gluten sensitivity."

Likewise, numerous parents report that their children with various disorders (like eczema, colic, or acne) get better when milk is excluded from their diet. Perhaps similar mechanisms are involved. This is of course controversial and only time will tell.

EFFECT ON SURVIVAL

It is one thing to look at effects on chronic ailments, it is another to take a global perspective and look at the effect on overall survival. Elwood and colleagues from The

University of Reading, U.K. conducted a meta-analysis of 14 cohort studies that demonstrated that in the backdrop of effects on diabetes, vascular disease and cancer, consumption of milk and dairy intake offers a survival advantage.

HEALTH CONSIDERATIONS BEYOND CONSUMING COW'S MILK

Long-term milking of cows increases the risk of breast infections like mastitis requiring antibiotics for treatment. Low levels of antibiotics can also be detected in milk that we consume.

Such antibiotic exposure in the gut can alter the gut flora, affecting the whole body, especially the immune system. In addition, this contributes to a rise in drug resistant bacteria, which can afflict us just like any other animals. Besides the possible effects on health, the frequent use of antibiotics in cattle also has potential for potentiating the problem of antibiotic resistant bacteria.

References

1. Lucassen P. Colic in infants. *BMJ Clin Evid*. 2010 Feb 5;2010. pii: 0309.

2. Hall B, Chesters J, Robinson A. Infantile colic: a systematic review of medical and conventional therapies. *J Paediatr Child Health*. 2012 Feb;48(2):128-37.

3. Uijterschout L, Vloemans J, Vos R et al. Prevalence and Risk Factors of Iron Deficiency in Healthy Young Children in the Southwestern Region of the Netherlands. *J Pediatr Gastroenterol Nutr*. 2013 Oct 17.

4. Arvola T, Ruuska T, Keränen J, Hyöty H, Salminen S, Isolauri E. Rectal bleeding in infancy: clinical, allergological, and microbiological examination. *Pediatrics*. 2006 Apr; 117(4):e760-8.

5. Monti G, Viola S, Baro C, Cresi F, Tovo PA et al. Tolerability of donkey's milk in 92 highly-problematic cow's milk allergic children. *J Biol Regul Homeost Agents*. 2012 Jul-Sep;26(3 Suppl):75-82.

6. Grulee C.G., and Sanford H.N.: The influence of breast and artificial feeding on infantile eczema. *J Pediatr* 1936; 9: pp. 223-225.

7. Jin Y.Y., Cao R.M., Chen J., et al: Partially hydrolyzed cow's milk formula has a therapeutic effect on the infants with mild to moderate atopic dermatitis: a randomized, double-blind study. *Pediatr Allergy Immunol* 2011; 22: pp. 688-694

8. Gdalevich M., Mimouni D., David M., and Minouni M.: Breastfeeding and the onset of atopic dermatitis in childhood: a systemic review and meta- analysis of prospective studies. *J Am Acad Dermatol* 2001; 45: pp. 520-527.

9. Sozańska B, Pearce N, Dudek K, Cullinan P. Consumption of unpasteurized milk and its effects on atopy and asthma in children and adult inhabitants in rural Poland. *Allergy*. 2013; 68(5):644-50.

10. Sackesen C, Assa'ad A, Baena-Cagnani C et al. Cow's milk allergy as a global

challenge. *Curr Opin Allergy Clin Immunol*. 2011 Jun; 11(3):243-8.

11. Maskatia ZK, Davis CM. Perinatal environmental influences on goat's and sheep's milk allergy without cow's milk allergy. *Ann Allergy Asthma Immunol*. 2013 Dec; 111(6):574-

12. Kull I., Bohme M., Wahlgren C.F., Nordvall L., Pershagen G., Wickman M. Breastfeeding reduces the risk for childhood eczema. *J Allergy Clin Immunol* 2005; 116: pp. 657-661.

13. Fleischer DM, Spergel JM, Assa'ad AH, Pongracic JA. Primary prevention of allergic disease through nutritional interventions. *J Allergy Clin Immunol Pract*. 2013 Jan; 1(1):29-36.

14. von Berg A., Filipiak-Pittroff B., Krämer U., et al: Preventive effect of hydrolyzed infant formulas persists until age 6 years: long-term results from the German Infant Nutritional Intervention Study (GINI). *J Allergy Clin Immunol* 2008; 121: pp. 1442-1447.

15. Kagalwalla AF, Amsden K, Shah A et al. Cow's milk elimination: a novel dietary approach to treat eosinophilic esophagitis. *J Pediatr Gastroenterol Nutr*. 2012 Dec; 55(6):711-6.

16. Topal E, Eğritaş O, Arga M et al. Eosinophilic esophagitis and anaphylaxis due to cow's milk in an infant. *Turk J Pediatr*. 2013 Mar-Apr; 55(2):222-5.

17. Hak E, de Vries TW, Hoekstra PJ, Jick SS. Association of childhood attention-deficit/hyperactivity disorder with atopic diseases and skin infections? A matched case-control study using the General Practice Research Database. *Ann Allergy Asthma Immunol*. 2013 Aug; 111(2):102-106.

18. Melnik BC, John SM, Schmitz G. Milk is not just food but most likely a genetic transfection system activating mTORC1 signaling for postnatal growth. *Nutr J*. 2013 Jul 25;12:103.

19. Adebamowo CA, Spiegelman D, Danby FW et al. High school dietary dairy intake

and teenage acne. *J Am Acad Dermatol*. 2005

20. Silverberg NB. Whey protein precipitating moderate to severe acne flares in 5 teenaged athletes. *Cutis*. 2012 Aug;90(2):70-2.

21. Mølgaard C, Larnkjær A, Arnberg K et al. Milk and growth in children: effects of whey and casein. *Nestle Nutr Workshop Ser Pediatr Program.* 2011;67:67-78.

22. Thorsdottir I, Thorisdottir AV. Whole cow's milk in early life. *Nestle Nutr Workshop Ser Pediatr Program.* 2011;67:29-40.

23. Griebler U, Bruckmüller MU, Kien C, Dieminger B et a. Health effects of cow's milk consumption in infants up to 3 years of age: a systematic review and meta-analysis. *Public Health Nutr*. 2015 May 20:1-15.

24. Patelarou E, Girvalaki C, Brokalaki H et al. Current evidence on the associations of breastfeeding, infant formula, and cow's milk introduction with type 1 diabetes

mellitus: a systematic review. *Nutr Rev.* 2012 Sep; 70(9):509-19.

25. Egro FM. Why is type 1 diabetes increasing? *J Mol Endocrinol.* 2013 Jul 12;51(1):R1-13.

26. Luopajärvi K, Savilahti E, Virtanen SM, et al. Enhanced levels of cow's milk antibodies in infancy in children who develop type 1 diabetes later in childhood. *Pediatr Diabetes.* 2008;9:434–441.

27. Kamal Alanani NM, Alsulaimani AA. Epidemiological pattern of newly diagnosed children with type 1 diabetes mellitus, taif, Saudi Arabia. *Scientific World Journal.* 2013 Oct 9; 2013: 421569.

28. Knip M, Virtanen SM, Seppä K, Ilonen J, Savilahti E et al. Finnish TRIGR Study Group. Dietary intervention in infancy and later signs of beta-cell autoimmunity. *N Engl J Med.* 2010 Nov 11;363(20):1900-8.

29. Gao D, Ning N, Wang C et al. Dairy products consumption and risk of type 2 diabetes: systematic review and dose-

response meta-analysis. *PLoS One*. 2013
Sep 27;8(9):e73965.

30. Chen M, Sun Q, Giovannucci E,
Mozaffarian D et al. Dairy consumption
and risk of type 2 diabetes: 3 cohorts of
US adults and an updated meta-analysis.
BMC Med. 2014 Nov 25;12:215.

31. Hu FB, Stampfer MJ, Manson JE et al.
Dietary saturated fats and their food
sources in relation to the risk of coronary
heart disease in women. *Am J Clin Nutr*.
1999 Dec;70(6):1001-8.

32. Larsson SC, Männistö S, Virtanen MJ et al.
Dairy foods and risk of stroke.
Epidemiology. 2009 May;20(3):355-60.

33. Kondo I, Ojima T, Nakamura M et al. and
NIPPON DATA80 Research Group.
Consumption of dairy products and death
from cardiovascular disease in the
Japanese general population: the NIPPON
DATA80. *J Epidemiol*. 2013;23(1):47-54.

34. Praagman J, Franco OH, Ikram MA et al.
Dairy products and the risk of stroke and

coronary heart disease: the Rotterdam Study. Eur J Nutr. 2014 Oct 9.

35. Jiang W, Ju C, Jiang H, Zhang D. Dairy foods intake and risk of Parkinson's disease: a dose-response meta-analysis of prospective cohort studies. *Eur J Epidemiol.* 2014 Sep;29(9):613-9.

36. Kistner A, Krack P. Parkinson's disease: no milk today? *Front Neurol.* 2014 Sep 5;5:172.

37. Whitley C, Gunst K, Müller H et al. Novel replication-competent circular DNA molecules from healthy cattle serum and milk and multiple sclerosis-affected human brain tissue. *Genome Announc.* 2014 Aug 28;2(4).

38. Murphy N, Norat T, Ferrari P et al. Consumption of dairy products and colorectal cancer in the European Prospective Investigation into Cancer and Nutrition (EPIC). *PLoS One.* 2013 Sep 2;8(9):e72715.

39. Abbastabar H, Roustazadeh A, Alizadeh A et al. Relationships of colorectal cancer

with dietary factors and public health indicators: an ecological study. *Asian Pac J Cancer Prev.* 2015;16(9):3991-5.

40. Aune D, Navarro Rosenblatt DA, Chan DS et al. Dairy products, calcium, and prostate cancer risk: a systematic review and meta-analysis of cohort studies. *Am J Clin Nutr.* 2015 Jan;101(1):87-117.

41. Tian SB, Yu JC, Kang WM, Ma ZQ, Ye X, Cao ZJ. Association between dairy intake and gastric cancer: a meta-analysis of observational studies. *PLoS One.* 2014 Jul 9;9(7):e101728.

42. Genkinger JM, Hunter DJ, Spiegelman D, et al. Dairy products and ovarian cancer: a pooled analysis of 12 cohort studies. *Cancer Epidemiol Biomarkers Prev* 2006; 15:364

43. Newcomb PA, Egan KM. Dairy food and ovarian cancer risk. *Lancet* 2006; 367:797.

44. Dong JY, Zhang L, He K, Qin LQ. Dairy consumption and risk of breast cancer: a meta-analysis of prospective cohort studies. *Breast Cancer Res Treat.* 2011

May;127(1):23-31. doi: 10.1007/s10549-011-1467-5.

45. Ji J, Sundquist J, Sundquist K. Lactose intolerance and risk of lung, breast and ovarian cancers: aetiological clues from a population-based study in Sweden. *Br J Cancer*. 2015 Jan 6;112(1):149-52.

46. Elwood PC, Givens DI, Beswick AD et al. The survival advantage of milk and dairy consumption: an overview of evidence from cohort studies of vascular diseases, diabetes and cancer. *J Am Coll Nutr*. 2008 Dec;27(6):723S-34S.

Section IV
Making Sense of Conflicting Information

CHAPTER 12

How Can Cow's Milk Cause Harm Only to Certain People?

TRANSFER OF COW'S GENETIC MATERIAL VIA MILK

Milk contains chemicals that contain sensitive genetic information. When consuming another animal's product, potentially coded and critical genetic information can be passed from the producer to the consumer – in this case, from cow to the human. Such transfer of genetic codes may bring about metabolic and immune transformation that could be useful or harmful; in some cases, it may be beneficial to the producer while being harmful to the consumer of the milk.

ROLE OF CASEIN PROTEINS IN MILK

We know that the casein in milk is digested into a variety of smaller chemicals or peptides with real biological actions. These smaller peptides when absorbed through the gut barrier, gain access to the brain and are capable of attaching to the morphine-like opioid binding areas in the brain. This can result in functional changes in the signalling and messaging link network in the nervous system.

This is not just a wild theory.

- Studies of milk have documented opioids occurring freely, as well as bound to other substances in the milk. This is just one example of an external influence of one species (cow) on the other (human).

- Commercially available synthetic casein breakdown products are widely used as an opioid tool for research purposes. They turn on the opioid binding sites in brain. Much of the data for the functional role for casein byproducts pertains to beta-casomorphins.

- The antibodies against cow's caseins are increased in patients with schizophrenia.

- Actions and interactions of casein breakdown products result in their actions as "food hormones" in the body, especially during infancy and early childhood. These interactions can sometimes be transformational and may theoretically alter the brain function and even reset brain function to a "new normal."

According to Dr. Roncada and colleagues from Italy, there may be a dormant biologic or metabolic activity that becomes unmasked when the large complex proteins like caseins are broken down into smaller peptides.

One factor that determines the adverse effects of any toxic substance is the total amount of toxin. The human body is able to handle breast milk with low casein proteins for a short time during infancy.

However, depending upon genetic predilection, the human body may not be able to handle a constant bombardment of a toxic substance (like caseins from cow's milk) day after day for the rest of the person's life.

This is especially so if the toxic barrage starts during the vulnerable formative years of childhood. This is even more likely if the early exposure is in the absence of potentially protective metabolic substances in human milk.

Consistent with this theory, studies from Dr. Nakamura's laboratory have demonstrated that consuming pre-digested casein in lieu of whole casein protein increases work efficiency, stabilizes brain activity, and reduces anxiety.

THINK EPIGENETICS!

It should be noted that milk is most likely not the sole culprit for a disease when it occurs. It likely acts in conjunction with other insults whose combined onslaught forms a larger insult and causes damage.

Other insults may include living in areas exposed to high traffic or pollution, eating a high-gluten diet, and consuming meat from animals exposed to pesticides and contaminated with antibiotics.

POTENTIAL IMPACT OF CONTINUED MILK CONSUMPTION

Mother's milk is not just critical for the brain. Babies that are not breastfed are usually fed cow's milk-based formula. However, this strategy may increase the long-term risk of a variety of diseases in a subset of genetically vulnerable people.

Humans are the only species that consume milk past infancy. The continued lifetime exposure to very high concentrations of casein of cow's proteins has the potential to cause continued and worsening damage in those vulnerable to such toxicity. And, of course, the ability to digest lactose declines past childhood and has its own potential for problems.

Breastfed and formula-fed babies have a different growth curve, frequency of infections, and a variable risk for many diseases, like celiac disease, diabetes, obesity, hypertension, allergies, high cholesterol and cancer. Lack of breastfeeding has also been implicated in the causation of inflammatory bowel disease and autism.

A recent systematic review by Pereira and colleagues concluded that the absence of breastfeeding is a modifiable risk factor for the development of diabetes. Breastfeeding is of benefit to moms as well. It reduces the risk of breast cancer!

REFERENCES

1. Roncada P, Stipetic LH, Bonizzi L et al. Proteomics as a tool to explore human milk in health and disease. *J Proteomics*. 2013 Aug 2;88:47-57.

2. Dohan FC. Genetic hypothesis of idiopathic schizophrenia: its exorphin connection. *Schizophr Bull*. 1988; 14(4):489-94.

3. Pereira PF, Alfenas Rde C, Araújo RM. Does breastfeeding influence the risk of developing diabetes mellitus in children? A review of current evidence. *J Pediatr* (Rio J). 2014 Jan-Feb;90(1):7-15.

CHAPTER 13

Is it Leaky Gut?

The trouble with the world is that the stupid are cocksure and the intelligent full of doubt.

---Bertrand Russell

Gut is not a wall of concrete and is always porous or leaky. After all, it has to let the essential nutrients, medications etc. across the intestinal wall and into the body.

INTESTINAL BARRIER

The intestinal barrier is like a chain-link fence. The joints of the chain links of the barrier are known as "tight junctions." These junctions are not absolutely tight. Rather, they are meant to be selective, i.e. they open up to allow food and other beneficial substances to go across the gut wall into the body. At the same time, they close ranks literally to keep the harmful materials and bacteria at bay.

While "leaky gut" is a fact, the term and the concept of "leaky gut syndrome" is controversial. Many in mainstream medicine reject the idea. On the other hand, most integrative physicians and nutritionists are big proponents and recommend strategies to strengthen the intestinal barrier. Pharmaceutical companies are working hard to develop drugs to heal abnormal "tight junctions" of the barrier seen in many diseases.

UNHEALTHY BACTERIAL BALANCE AND LEAKY GUT

EXAMPLE OF UNHEALTHY GUT BACTERIA

An imbalance of gut bacteria in favor of harmful inflammatory bacteria like *Clostridia* and *Desulfovibrio* at the expense of anti-inflammatory bacteria of *Bifidobacteria* type can sometimes occur and is unhealthy. This is known as dysbiosis and has been implicated in the pathogenesis of numerous disorders including neurobehavioral dysfunctions like autism.

WHAT HAPPENS IN LEAKY GUT?

The altered bacterial balance in favor of increased inflammation results in leaky gut. There is widening or loosening of the "tight junctions" of this gut barrier allowing passage of toxins, including brain-toxic compounds into the body. These neuro-toxic compounds may be derived from dietary components or the unhealthy bacteria themselves. They can cause inflammation in the brain resulting in neuro-behavioral problems including possibly autism. The variation in behavioral problems may vary with the type of toxin as well as the part of brain affected by the toxin.

AGENT-BASED MODEL FOR UNHEALTHY GUT IN AUTISM

An agent-based modeling framework has been developed by Dr. Weston and colleagues from the University of Delaware. It demonstrates that any intrusion or distraction such as the use of prebiotics or antibiotics have only a transient effect on bacterial balance.

On the other hand, prolonged prebiotic intake may enhance the low populations of beneficial *Bifidobacteria*. Similarly, frequent antibiotic use may help sustain bad unhealthy bacteria. Furthermore, their simulations indicate that the growth rate of the bad *Clostridia bacteria* is a key element which impacts on the risk of developing autism.

Treatment of high-risk infants with supra-physiological levels of lysozymes may suppress clostridia growth rate, resulting in a steep decrease in the clostridia population and therefore a reduced risk of autism development. Their simulations also suggest that the number of clostridia bacteria plays a critical role in development of autism.

DO STUDIES INDICATE POSSIBLE BENEFIT FROM PROBIOTICS?

According to Dr. Mayer and colleagues from the Oppenheimer Center for Neurobiology of Stress at UCLA in Los Angeles, CA, an animal model of autism involving maternal infection demonstrates neurobehavioral changes associated with intestinal changes including altered gut bacterial profile. This *"suggests a possible benefit of probiotic treatment on several of the observed abnormal behaviors."*

COW'S MILK AND LEAKY GUT LINK

In contrast to the human milk, the cow's milk has different types as well as higher levels of casein proteins. The metabolic breakdown products of some caseins have the potential to adversely affect the brain if they can get absorbed through the gut and eventually gain access to the brain.

Adverse effects have been documented in laboratory studies. "Tight junctions" do not live up to their name in the presence of leaky gut and the chain link fence has wider holes. The abnormally porous leaky gut thus facilitates the passage of the potentially neuro-toxic breakdown products of cow's milk casein.

As noted earlier, cow's milk is most likely not the sole offending factor in the development of most situations. Results from the *ScanBrit trial* demonstrated benefits from a gluten-free, casein-free diet in subjects with autism lending support to the above concept.

Variable results from casein-free diet studies led Dr. van De Sande and colleagues from the Nutrition, Toxicology and Metabolism Research Institute in Maastricht, The Netherlands, to conclude that *"nutrition and other environmental influences might trigger an unstable base of genetic predisposition, which may lead to the development of autism…"*

The American Academy of Pediatrics has recommended more research into the role of gut, digestion and nutrition in autism spectrum disorders.

STRENGTHENING THE LEAKY GUT MAY HELP

Unfortunately there are no well-established drugs that heal intestinal hyper-permeability or leaky gut exclusively. Some of the drugs healing chronic inflammatory disorders like rheumatoid arthritis, ulcerative colitis and Crohn's disease do reduce the intestinal permeability.

Drug companies are working fast and furious to develop pharmaceutical options. Recently, one pharmaceutical agent called larazotide has been demonstrated to relieve symptoms of celiac disease, a classic example of leaky gut, without implementing a gluten-free diet!

Larazotide blocks the opening of tight junctions. Dr. Kelly and colleagues from the Harvard Medical School in Boston, MA, conducted a double-blind, randomized, placebo-controlled trial of 184 patients previously on a gluten-free diet. Subjects were randomized to receive larazotide or placebo plus 2.7 grams of gluten every day for 6 weeks.

The investigators documented that the celiac disease subjects taking larazotide had decreased gluten-induced symptoms despite consuming gluten. The traditional tests of gut leakiness were not affected suggesting that the currently available tests may not be sensitive enough.

While we await the advent of pharmaceutical remedies for leaky gut, patients may try non-pharmaceutical strategies like eating a healthy, well-balanced diet.

A detailed discussion of the topic of leaky gut is beyond the scope of this book and has been reviewed by many authors in literature. One of the available options on this topic is the book, "Is it Leaky Gut or Leaky Gut Syndrome" written by this author.

REFERENCES

1. Catassi C, Bonucci A, Coppa GV, et al. Intestinal permeability changes during the first month: effect of natural versus artificial feeding. *J Pediatr Gastroenterol Nutr.* 1995;21:383–386.

2. Nguyen DN, Li Y, Sangild PT, Bering SB, Chatterton DE. Effects of bovine lactoferrin on the immature porcine intestine. *Br J Nutr.* 2014 Jan 28;111(2):321-31.

3. Leffler DA, Kelly CP, Green PH et al. Larazotide acetate for persistent symptoms of celiac disease despite a gluten-free diet: a randomized controlled trial. *Gastroenterology.* 2015 Jun;148(7):1311-1319.

4. Weston B, Fogal B, Cook D, Dhurjati P. An agent-based modeling framework for evaluating hypotheses on risks for

developing autism: effects of the gut microbial environment. *Med Hypotheses.* 2015 Apr;84(4):395-401.

5. Vaarala O. Is it dietary insulin? *Ann N Y Acad Sci.* 2006 Oct;1079:350-9.

6. Kalach N, Rocchiccioli F, de Boissieu D, Benhamou PH, Dupont C. Intestinal permeability in children: variation with age and reliability in the diagnosis of cow's milk allergy. *Acta Paediatr.* 2001 May;90(5):499-504.

7. Terpend K, Blaton MA, Candalh C et al. Intestinal barrier function and cow's milk sensitization in guinea pigs fed milk or fermented milk. *J Pediatr Gastroenterol Nutr.* 1999 Feb;28(2):191-8.

8. Darmon N, Abdoul E, Roucayrol AM, Blaton MA et al. Sensitization to cow's milk proteins during refeeding of guinea pigs recovering from polydeficient malnutrition. *Pediatr Res.* 1998 Dec;44(6):931-8.

9. Mayer EA, Padua D, Tillisch K. Altered brain-gut axis in autism: comorbidity or

causative mechanisms? *Bioessays*. 2014 Oct;36(10):933-9.

10. van De Sande MM, van Buul VJ, Brouns FJ. Autism and nutrition: the role of the gut-brain axis. *Nutr Res Rev.* 2014 Dec;27(2):199-214.

CHAPTER 14

Milk Banks

Most of us know that breast milk feeding helps the baby in part by enhancing immunity to fight infections. In the preceding chapters, we have discussed the role of breast feeding and cow's milk on the short and long term health of the child.

Breast milk feeding also results in improved cognitive function or a brainy child! What parent would not want that!

Caution: Breastfed infants should receive vitamin D supplementation.

In cases of infants weaned prior to the age of 1 year, an iron-fortified infant formula and not just cow's milk should be used.

CONTRAINDICATIONS OF BREAST FEEDING

Breastfeeding may not be appropriate in a few select situations.

- Galactose 1-phosphate uridyltransferase deficiency.

- Maternal infections can be a big factor if not addressed. These include active untreated tuberculosis, varicella infection etc. Breast feeding in the presence of maternal hepatitis may be ok in the setting of adequate immune prophylaxis.

- Mothers receiving radiation therapy.

- Mothers receiving chemotherapy for cancer.

- Mothers with HIV or AIDS.

- Mothers using street/recreational drugs.

- Mothers with Herpes simplex lesions on a breast. However, if only one breast is affected, feeding may be accomplished from the other without lesions.

If breast milk is not an option, milk obtained from milk banks is the next best option.

MILK BANKS IN LIEU OF BREAST FEEDING

Just as the breastfeeding of babies by lactating mothers has been gaining in popularity, so is the use of milk banks by moms unable to breastfeed. However, availability of milk banks also has the potential to undermine the concept and policy of breastfeeding.

In the case of specialized at-risk children, like pre-term babies, neither the donor human milk nor the usual formula milk can meet the total nutritional needs and as such fortification is required.

According to Dr. Miracle and colleagues from Rush University in Chicago, IL, key ethical issues involve *"medical decision-making and informed consent, increasing the limited supply of human milk, how ethically to allocate this scarce resource, and concerns linked to the marketing of a human milk."*

USE OF DONOR MILK FROM MILK BANKS

Human milk may be obtained from a milk bank in cases where mothers are unable to breastfeed the baby. In case of premature babies, the quantity of nutrients in breast milk may not meet the heightened nutrient needs.

Donor pasteurized human milk may serve as a useful proxy for the mother's own milk. Human milk supplements, or fortifiers, may be used to supplement the nutrient content of unfortified breast milk. Host defense benefits are also observed in such situations.

MILK BANK GUIDELINES

In order to maximize the benefits and minimize the risks of donated milk from milk banks, strict guidelines have been set forth by the Human Milk Bank of North America. While local regulations may vary, these generally include the following:

- Donors of milk are screened by clinical history and blood tests to exclude HIV, hepatitis B and C, HTLV and syphilis.

- Milk is collected, pooled and pasteurized.

- Creamatocrit is also performed to determine the calorie/nutrient content.

ALL MILK BANKS ARE NOT THE SAME

Landers and colleagues point out the different practices involving milk banks in different parts of the world and *"the differing criteria for donor selection, current pasteurization techniques, and quality control measures."*

EFFECT OF PASTEURIZATION

Pasteurization of donor milk results in killing of several viruses with only a limited impact on antibodies, growth factors, lysozyme etc. However, microwaving does significantly destroy the anti-infective components in the milk.

Note that no GVHD (graft versus host disease) occurs as a result of milk therapy.

REFERENCES

1. Miracle DJ, Szucs KA, Torke AM, Helft PR. Contemporary ethical issues in human milk-banking in the United States. *Pediatrics*. 2011 Dec;128(6):1186-91.

2. Jones F. Milk sharing: how it undermines breastfeeding. *Breastfeed Rev.* 2013Nov;21(3):21-5.

3. Simmer K. The knowns and unknowns of human milk banking. *Nestle Nutr Workshop Ser Pediatr Program*. 2011;68:49-61; discussion 61-4.

4. Centre for Clinical Practice at NICE (UK). Donor Breast Milk Banks: The Operation of Donor Milk Bank Services. London: *National Institute for Health and Clinical Excellence (UK)*; 2010 Feb.

5. ESPGHAN Committee on Nutrition, Arslanoglu S, Corpeleijn W, Moro G, Braegger C et al. Donor human milk for preterm infants: current evidence and research directions. J Pediatr Gastroenterol Nutr. 2013 Oct;57(4):535-42.

6. Landers S, Hartmann BT. Donor human milk banking and the emergence of milk sharing. *Pediatr Clin North Am*. 2013 Feb;60(1):247-60.

7. Brent N. The risks and benefits of human donor breast milk. *Pediatr Ann*. 2013 May;42(5):84-90.

CHAPTER 15

Concluding Thoughts

Do not fear to be eccentric in opinion, for every opinion now accepted was once eccentric.

---Bertrand Russell

MILK IS NOT THE PROBLEM, IT'S WHERE IT COMES FROM

In contrast to cow's milk that is homogenized and pasteurized, human milk is uniquely constructed to meet a human baby's needs. Mom's milk for the baby provides highly individualized nutrition for the growing baby based on the stage of infancy. In addition, it provides bioactive immune-beneficial compounds.

Each human's milk can be different from the next, based on the changing needs of the baby, while the cow's milk stays same.

The importance of proper nutrition in early life is highlighted by the fact that premature infants need dietary quality more than quantity for optimal growth and development. Studies suggest that the dietary pattern during infancy and early childhood affects development of brain.

Since human milk is just produced for one baby, it is produced in smaller amounts, usually about 600-900 ml per day. In contrast, cow's milk is produced in large quantities for bulk consumption.

Cow's milk varies a lot as well depending upon breed. For example, most milk in U.S. and Europe comes from one particular breed.

Selective breeding has potential for generating milk whose breakdown products can be more toxic than others especially when compared to milk derived from cows freely grazing in pastures and without exposure to pollutants, toxins, artificial feeds and unnecessary antibiotics.

IS MILK TOTALLY BAD?

Milk is not bad. Infants should drink milk, preferably their mother's milk, and then be weaned off.

YOU ARE HEALTHY UNTIL YOU ARE UNHEALTHY

The problem is that it is difficult to clearly define who may be at risk or benefit from inclusion of cow's milk before a disorder occurs. Even then, literature-based evidence on problems related to cow's milk is mostly circumstantial.

At the same time, it is hard to ignore the fact that cow's milk has been a boon for preventing malnutrition, especially in developing countries. Until more hard data is available, the debate will continue to be opinion-based and passionate.

THE CHOICE IS YOURS

WHO DOES IT AFFECT?

It's your child's body, and your child's brain.

It affects you as well. It's your body, both over short and long term.

THINK HARD

Bertrand Russell once stated, *"The most savage controversies are those about matters as to which there is no good evidence either way."*

There may not be a single perfect answer. There may not be a single answer that fits all. There may be one answer for populations in poor developing countries being fed cow's milk from genetically unselected cows grazing freely without exposure to any toxic chemicals or unnecessary antibiotics.

The answer may be different for well off and at risk people in developed countries being fed milk from cows constantly constrained in close quarters, exposed to a variety of potentially toxic chemicals or antibiotics or both and genetically selected for the sole purpose of increased milk production without regard for the higher levels of potentially toxic, biologically-active components in the milk.

Everyone will interpret the data differently. One fact remains constant. The medical science and knowledge continues to evolve fast and furious. The questions raised in this book and possible answers are unlikely to remain the same in future.

I am one with *Socrates* when he said, "*I am the wisest man alive, and that is that I know nothing.*"

Knowledge is power. Do your own due diligence!

DR. MINOCHA'S PLEA

Irrespective of the conclusions you may draw from reading this book and the strategy you adopt for yourself and your child, please don't judge anyone else for making a decision that may be different than yours. Everyone's situation is different. Don't forget, the final word on this issue is probably yet to be written. Only God knows the final answer and He has not spoken to me. At least not yet.

HEALTH IS WEALTH.

May God bless you and all those around you with the best of health.

Bonus Section

Sneak Peak at Other Books

by Dr. Minocha

CHAPTER I

Select Listing of Diseases Linked to Leaky Gut

Below is chapter #10 from Dr. Minocha' book, "Is it Leaky Gut or Leaky Gut Syndrome."

KEY POINTS

- Leaky gut is associated with a wide variety of disorders involving diverse organ systems of the body.

- Many of these diseases tend to co-occur in the same individual.

Interpreting Tests for Leaky Gut

This book cites numerous studies documenting abnormalities on tests for intestinal permeability. Consider those tests in proper context. Bear in mind that most available tests for leaky gut are rudimentary.

None of the available tests can investigate all the possible pathways whereby noxious substances can cross between the adjacent cells and/or directly through the cells of the gut barrier. Available tests do not also test for passage of fat soluble substances.

SELECT LISTING

GI DISEASES

- Celiac disease

- Crohn's disease

- Ulcerative colitis

- Irritable bowel syndrome

- Collagenous colitis

- Gastrointestinal infections

- NSAID enteropathy (GI problems due to aspirin-like drugs)

- Chemotherapy-induced gut injury

- Pseudomembranous colitis

ENDOCRINE DISEASES

- Diabetes mellitus

- Autoimmune thyroiditis

- Obesity and metabolic syndrome

ALLERGIC DISORDERS

- Food allergies

- Skin eczema

- Asthma

- Nasal allergies

BACTERIAL INFECTIONS

- Cholera

- Helicobacter pylori in stomach

- Clostridium perfringens

- Clostridium difficile

- Certain forms of E. coli

VIRAL INFECTIONS

- Adenovirus

- Cox-Sackie virus

- Rotavirus

- HIV

- Hepatitis C

SKIN DISEASES

- Acne

- Psoriasis

- Rosacea

- Urticaria

LIVER DISEASES

- Alcoholic liver disease

- Intrahepatic cholestasis of pregnancy

- Nonalcoholic fatty liver disease

- Primary biliary cirrhosis

- Primary sclerosing cholangitis

RHEUMATOLOGICAL DISEASES

- Rheumatoid arthritis

- Lupus

- Ankylosing spondylitis

VASCULAR (BLOOD VESSELS) SYSTEM

- Edema or fluid swelling

- Endotoxemia

- Retinal complications of diabetes

- Hematogenous (blood-borne) spread of cancer

NEURO-PSYCHO-BEHAVIORAL DYSFUNCTION

- Emotional stress

- Autism

- Schizophrenia

- Depression

CHRONIC PAIN SYNDROMES

- Fibromyalgia

- Chronic fatigue syndrome

NEUROLOGICAL DISORDERS

- Multiple sclerosis

- Chronic inflammatory demyelinating polyneuropathy

- Parkinson's disease

MISCELLANEOUS

- Heart failure

- Parenteral or intravenous nutrition (Fasting patient obtaining nutrition via veins)

- Multi-organ failure

- Graft versus host disease

- Cancer and it's spread locally and metastasis to distant organs

REFERENCES

1. Zhang L, Cheng J, Fan XM. MicroRNAs: New therapeutic targets for intestinal

barrier dysfunction. *World J Gastroenterol.* 2014 May 21;20(19):5818-5825.

2. de Punder K, Pruimboom L. The dietary intake of wheat and other cereal grains and their role in inflammation. *Nutrients.* 2013 Mar 12;5(3):771-87.

3. Lu Z, Ding L, Lu Q, Chen YH. Claudins in intestines: Distribution and functional significance in health and diseases. *Tissue Barriers.* 2013 Jul 1;1(3):e24978.

4. Ding L, Lu Z, Lu Q, Chen YH. The claudin family of proteins in human malignancy: a clinical perspective. *Cancer Manag Res.* 2013 Nov 8;5:367-75.

5. Fries W, Belvedere A, Vetrano S. Sealing the broken barrier in IBD: intestinal permeability, epithelial cells and junctions. *Curr Drug Targets.* 2013 Nov;14(12):1460-70.

6. Sawada N. Tight junction-related human diseases. *Pathol Int.* 2013 Jan;63(1):1-12.

7. Catalioto RM, Maggi CA, Giuliani S. Intestinal epithelial barrier dysfunction in

disease and possible therapeutical interventions. *Curr Med Chem*. 2011;18(3):398-426.

8. Caricilli AM, Castoldi A, Câmara NO. Intestinal barrier: A gentlemen's agreement between microbiota and immunity. *World J Gastrointest Pathophysiol*. 2014 Feb 15;5(1):18-32.

9. Price DB, Ackland ML, Burks W et al. Peanut Allergens Alter Intestinal Barrier Permeability and Tight Junction Localisation in Caco-2 Cell Cultures. *Cell Physiol Biochem*. 2014 May 23;33(6):1758-1777.

Overview of Dr. M's Seven-X Plan

Below is chapter #42 from Dr. Minocha's book, "Dr. M's Seven-X Plan for Digestive Health."

KEY POINTS

- You are healthy until you are unhealthy.

- Using the Seven-X Plan for healing is good – adopting it for prevention is even better.

Now is the time when rubber hits the road. You have presumably gone through the background material I have provided in the previous chapters. And I am sure most of you already have a pretty good idea of the health problems you face, the things that might be doing wrong, all the challenges you face, and the opportunities for improvement.

In a nutshell, there are some core elements of the program that everyone needs to adopt. And then there are some specific modifiable elements. The latter pertain to the specific type of nutrition based on your genetically-engineered and environmentally-transformed intestinal metabolic constitution.

My goal thus far in the book has been to empower you with knowledge so you may judge for yourself what is good for you. Since the science is not advanced enough to test for it, we just have two main elements to guide us:

Overall health of the person and presence or absence of diverse illnesses.

Reaction of the person's body to any single food or the type of foods – for example, most people with lactose intolerance can easily handle one glass of milk per day especially if consumed in split doses. However, a person with irritable bowel syndrome may not be able to tolerate even that.

So who are the candidates for Dr. M's Seven-X Plan? Is it for everyone to some extent or just for those with perceived unhealthy digestion?

Let's just divide the readers into four broad categories.

Patients with an unhealthy gut, digestion problems like irritable bowel syndrome, chronic heartburn, etc.

Patients with multiple illnesses, where unhealthy gut might be one component related to the primary illness, such as GI problems in patients with diabetes.

Patients with neurobehavioral problems and chronic pain syndromes where GI symptoms may be present and the unhealthy gut may be playing a critical role in sustaining the pain and brain and gut dysfunction.

Ostensibly healthy persons who look and feel great and of whom many of us feel jealous.

PERSONS WITH AN UNHEALTHY GUT

Not much write-up is needed here to justify the need for such patients to follow the gut-healthy

Seven-X Plan. While following the general principles outlined in the succeeding chapters, the patient must take into account the information in previous chapters where I may have provided disease-specific information. This will allow the person to modify the Seven-X Plan specifically to the illness.

One example would be patients with IBS. Such patients would benefit from the use of specific probiotic strains targeted at IBS and mentioned in Chapter 37.

Another example is gastroparesis or slow stomach. There is not just a decreased ability to tolerate food, but patients may have many other associated problems, including but not limited to malabsorption of nutrients and overgrowth of bad bacteria in the gut. In cases of gastroparesis, unlike many other GI disorders, we frequently recommend a low-fiber diet! This is just one example of how one needs to modify the Seven-X Plan based on the individual GI disorders described earlier.

PERSONS WITH NON-GI PRIMARY
ILLNESS OR MULTIPLE ILLNESSES

Subjects with multiple bodily illnesses (such as diabetes and lupus) frequently have GI problems.

And if it is not due to some illness, the GI symptoms may also arise as a result of medications being used to treat the illness. You just have to look at the package insert of any of your medicines and you will find that GI side effects are almost always listed as a possibility.

Patients with such conditions develop unhealthy gut due to their primary disease or the medicine they are taking. For example, when diabetes is associated with leaky gut and inflammation as causative factors, the diabetes may result in slowing down the gut or cause diarrhea. Medications like NSAIDs can cause indigestion and even ulcers anywhere in the gut.

Side effects of many acid-blocking medicines include weakened absorption of nutritional elements, small intestinal bacterial overgrowth, and increased risk of infections, including GI and non-GI infections.

PERSONS WITH NEUROBEHAVIORAL AND CHRONIC PAIN SYNDROMES

Notwithstanding the fact that the majority of such patients have concurrent GI issues, an unhealthy gut is one of the critical elements at the root of the perceived main problem.

> GI problems are a significant part of life for the vast majority of such patients, whether the diagnosis is autism, ADHD, OCD or one of the chronic pain syndromes, like fibromyalgia, chronic fatigue syndrome, or restless leg syndrome.

The preceding chapters on intestinal bacteria, leaky gut, inflammation, and oxidative stress have gone into the rationale behind this assertion. Needless to say, a full-throated adoption of Dr. M's Seven-X Plan will likely help soothe the illness.

ARE THERE ANY "PERFECTLY" HEALTHY PERSONS

A person is only healthy until he or she becomes unhealthy. Dr. M's Seven-X Plan serves as an insurance policy that will help any hidden problems that might be lurking inside the bowels of our body (no pun intended).

Let me explain this with an example. Former President George W. Bush has always been fit as a fiddle and passed his physicals done by the best physicians with flying colors. He continued his strenuous exercise routine after leaving the White House. Then one day, he was admitted to the hospital, where in he was found to have a life-threatening blockage of his arteries of his heart. Obviously, this blockage did not arise overnight. All through the years, there had been no alarm bells of anything ominous going on. Had he not received prompt medical attention, he could have died.

Another example you might know: Former President Bill Clinton always looked great and had regular check-ups. Although he had an aggressive exercise routine, he was notorious for his love for fast food. Years after he left the White House, he had to be admitted to the hospital, where a critical blockage of his arteries in heart was found. He underwent emergency bypass surgery. Subsequently, he adopted a vegan lifestyle, lost his excess body weight, and continues to work on his Clinton Global Initiative. By the way, Mr. Clinton did not change his religion when he switched to a vegan lifestyle; he just did it for his health and feels proud of it. Obviously, Mr. Clinton was thinking on the lines of experts like Dr. Jane Ferguson from the Perelman School of Medicine at the University of Pennsylvania, who has written a report titled, "Meat-loving microbes: Do Steak-Eating Bacteria Promote Atherosclerosis?" She then goes on to provide evidence for an affirmative answer to this question.

A note of caution

One should not expect an overnight cure. Let perfection not be a barrier to good. A condition, perhaps with roots implanted in the womb and simmering for years, is unlikely to be reversed in short order. We need to be pragmatic. Patience is required! At the very least, based on what I know, I believe that Dr. M's Seven-X Plan will stem the downward slide of health and facilitate the body's natural processes to get on the path to mending.

The End

A PERSONAL NOTE FROM DR. MINOCHA

I truly appreciate you taking the time to read my thoughts on milk. If you liked the book, I would be extremely grateful if you would please show your love and support by writing a review for it on the amazon.com and goodreads.com websites.

Please tell the potential readers what you liked about the book and what you plan to do with the information. Your review would also help in my mission to share knowledge and promote health.

Thanks a million!

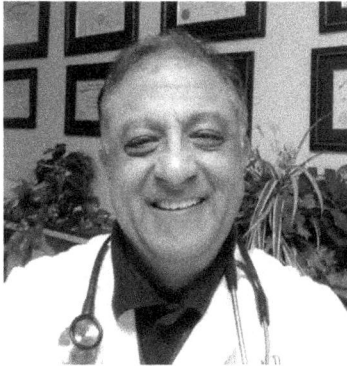

Anil Minocha MD

Facebook @doctoranil   Twitter @dranilminocha

DEDICATION

This book is dedicated to my family: my loving parents Ram and Kamla, my siblings Kamal, Vimal and Rina, and the light of my life Geeta. Without their unconditional love and support, this book would not have been possible.

PRAISE FOR "DR. M'S SEVEN-X PLAN FOR DIGESTIVE HEALTH"

"If you are looking for a holistic whole-body solution to your digestive ailments, then this is the book for you! "

---Dr. Robynne Chutkan, author of *Gutbliss*

"A treasure trove of key information on probiotics, intestinal infections and everything you ever could want to know about the digestive system."

---Chris Adamec, co-author of *Fibromyalgia for Dummies*

"I found the information on the role of bacteria in gut health as well as GI disease and dysfunction…very helpful and his description of his practical Seven-X Plan is easy to understand and follow."

--- Jill Sklar, author of *The First Year: Crohn's Disease and Ulcerative Colitis*

"If the proverbial 'cast iron' describes only other people's stomachs, you'll be fascinated by this accessible and infinitely helpful guide to your own GI system and how to keep it healthy."

--- Victoria Moran, author of *Main Street Vegan*